Praise for
# HIGH FIBER KETO

"Naomi Whittel has provided a deep dive into gaining a metabolic advantage through movement and a high fiber ketogenic diet. *High Fiber Keto*'s science-based plan describes six optimizers to enhance your metabolism and gain control of your body's energy source."

— **Mark Sisson**, founder of Primal Kitchen and *New York Times* best-selling author of *The Keto Reset Diet*

"If you're doing the keto diet, you're probably been doing it wrong. *High Fiber Keto* teaches you how to keep burning fat without losing the vital benefits of fiber. Read this book if you want to feel and look your best for the rest of your life."

— **Dave Asprey**, *New York Times* best-selling author of *Super Human*

"The accelerated popularity of high-fat ketogenic diets has created tremendous confusion around maintaining the important levels of plant compounds, fibers, and micro-nutrients. *High Fiber Keto* takes a science-based lifestyle-focused approach to utilizing all of the important plants to reap the benefits of natural medicine."

— **Dr. Josh Axe, DC, DNM, CNS**, co-founder of Ancient Nutrition and best-selling author of *Eat Dirt* and *Keto Diet*

"Sugar shrinks your brain and expands your waistline. While a ketogenic diet solves this problem, it also robs the digestive system of fiber. Naomi's program solves this by adding fiber to a ketogenic diet from a whole-foods perspective. Everyone seeking a healthy way to maintain nutritional ketosis should read this book."

— **Dr. Mike Dow**, *New York Times* best-selling author of *The Sugar Brain Fix*

"Naomi's new book *High Fiber Keto* addresses the most important factor essential for maximizing the benefits of the ketogenic diet, and that's incorporating the proper balance of specific high-fiber foods. This book covers the latest science and the proper implementation of what is the optimal ketogenic diet."

— **Dominic D'Agostino, Ph.D.**, associate professor at Morsani College of Medicine, University of South Florida

# HIGH

# FIBER

# KETO

# HIGH FIBER KETO

A 22-Day Science-Based Plan to
Fix Your Metabolism, Lose Weight,
and Balance Your Hormones

## NAOMI WHITTEL
with **Maryann Walsh**, M.F.N., R.D., C.D.E.

**HAY HOUSE, INC.**
Carlsbad, California • New York City
London • Sydney • New Delhi

*Published in the United States by:* Hay House, Inc.: www.hayhouse.com • *Published in Australia by:* Hay House Australia Pty. Ltd.: www.hay house.com.au • *Published in the United Kingdom by:* Hay House UK, Ltd.: www.hayhouse.co.uk • *Published in India by:* Hay House Publishers India: www.hayhouse.co.in

*Indexer:* Joan Shapiro
*Cover design:* Kathleen Lynch • *Interior design:* Nick C. Welch

**Cataloging-in-Publication Data is on file with the Library of Congress**

**Hardcover ISBN:** 978-1-4019-5887-9
**e-book ISBN:** 978-1-4019-5919-7
**Audiobook ISBN:** 978-1-4019-5935-7

10  9  8  7  6  5  4  3  2  1
1st edition, February 2020

Printed in the United States of America

SFI label applies to the text stock

This book is dedicated to my grandfather, and brilliant physicist, Jean-Paul Auffray, Ph.D. A man to whom I am eternally grateful. Not only for his love, but for his encouragement. As a little girl, he held my hand and guided me to embrace my curiosity and go off the beaten path, which has led to a better life.

# CONTENTS

# FOREWORD

Health and happiness go hand in hand for so many reasons, and because the foundation of health lies in your diet, it's safe to assume that a healthful diet mixed with exercise or movement that you enjoy can help make you happy in so many ways.

How much happier would you be with more energy, better metabolic health markers, and better feelings about your body and how your clothes fit? Better digestion? It's safe to say that most would feel happier!

Oftentimes we overlook the connection between our diet and how it affects our overall happiness, but I urge you to take a deep look into how your current dietary habits may be affecting your happiness day to day.

For thousands upon thousands of individuals, the ketogenic diet has been that one diet or way of eating that has just "stuck" for them. As a Registered Dietitian and Certified Diabetes Educator that specializes in weight loss, I have worked with so many wonderful clients who started off as "keto-curious." They had tried to lose weight or achieve better health through numerous other dietary plans, and they had heard so many talking about keto that they figured: why not give this a try? What have I got to lose? The often initial quick loss of body weight that many experience on keto is, of course, exciting, but it was the surprise of how wonderful they felt that kept them going. And the food? That is one of the best parts!

I always say that there has never been a better time to be following a ketogenic diet! There are a wealth of recipes and wonderful products on the market that make going keto incredibly delicious and incredibly convenient and easy.

I am beyond excited to be a part of *High Fiber Keto*. Naomi has done something that nobody else has been able to do so eloquently: take real, credible information from the top medical and scientific experts in the world on the topic of the ketogenic diet and assemble it into an easy-to-follow plan that includes delicious recipes and meal and snack suggestions that set you up for success.

As someone with a health and science background, it can be frustrating to see so much confusing information on the Internet, and more often than not it is released with the best of intentions. *High Fiber Keto* will save you time and effort in getting started on a ketogenic diet, because this book and this program takes the guesswork out of the process.

And what's one of my favorite parts of *High Fiber Keto*? The fact that this plan incorporates the health promoting, satiating power of fiber! Fiber not only promotes healthy digestion and helps to keep us full and satisfied, but a growing body of research is supporting the idea that prebiotic fiber, like inulin, helps support the tremendous role that our gut health plays in our mental health as well. So whether your goal is health, happiness, or to look and feel better, it's safe to say you hold an amazing wealth of knowledge in your hands right now to help you on your journey toward achieving these goals.

I wish you all the health and happiness you desire!

— Maryann Walsh, M.F.N., R.D., C.D.E.

# INTRODUCTION

Confident . . . compassionate . . . smart . . . determined.

These are a few of the words I would use to describe the amazing women I am so fortunate to know. Their collective strength, persistence, and passion for life can move mountains. They are wives, mothers, daughters, businesswomen, colleagues, friends, and much more. They work hard to never fail anyone they love.

And they succeed. We all succeed thanks to our strength and resilience. But there's always more to be done. We constantly struggle to have the energy to live up to our own expectations and those of every person who relies on us. Yet we always push ourselves to keep going because that's what we've always done, haven't we?

But sometimes there just isn't anything left in the tank, where we feel we have nothing left to give. Over time, our hectic schedules, stress, inadequate diets, and lack of sleep take their toll and do real damage to our bodies.

As a result, more than 100 million people in the U.S. have metabolic syndrome.[1] That's one-third of the country's entire population that suffers from at least three of the following: high blood pressure, high blood sugar, high levels of abdominal fat, a high triglyceride level, or a low HDL cholesterol level.

Millions more suffer from one or two of the risk factors, which makes them metabolically disadvantaged. By being metabolically disadvantaged or having metabolic syndrome, we put ourselves at risk for such conditions as chronic inflammation, hormone imbalance, heart disease, diabetes, and accelerated aging.

Recent research tells us that 75 percent of us, including me, are carb intolerant,[2] which means we should be using fat instead of carbohydrates as our primary fuel source. If we do, we can slow down and, in many cases, reverse the processes that cause these life-altering and life-limiting conditions. *High Fiber Keto* is the solution. My 22-day plan is the road map.

Because the ketogenic diet is low carb, unfortunately it can eliminate some of the precious fiber that we would normally gain through eating high-carbohydrate foods. As we know, fiber is necessary for good digestion, provides satiety, and can help prevent heart disease and diabetes.

My High Fiber Keto diet can solve that problem. This book is your guide to delicious foods that are nutrient dense and can help stave off metabolic syndrome and the myriad diseases that can result from it. A keto diet should include about 20 grams of fiber per day, but more than 90 percent of Americans don't reach that standard.

In my 20-plus-year career as a founder, wellness explorer, and CEO of health and well-being companies, I have guided millions of women to improve their lives through simple switches to their daily routine that have improved their health. Now I have developed my first lifestyle plan and method for optimizing and healing your metabolism to give you the strongest, leanest, and most beautiful version of you. Through the plan, you will learn about:

- The one ratio that reveals much more than the number on the scale

- The most efficient and effective form of fuel that will burn your own body fat

- New and delicious fiber-rich foods that will change the way your body looks and feels

- Pure, clean nutritional ingredients from around the world to help improve your body inside and out

- The most efficient and effective ways to move your body to ignite your metabolism

High Fiber Keto is a lifelong approach to losing and keeping off unnecessary and toxic fat, while developing your healthiest and most vibrant version of you. It all begins with reaching nutritional ketosis and working toward keto adaptation.

Here's what you can expect in these first 22 days:

*Body fat mass loss:* Up to 9.25 pounds

*Trimming of your waistline:* Lose up to 4 inches

*Rapid weight loss:* Lose up to 7 pounds

*Increased energy:* More alertness and focus during the day

*Beautiful, glowing skin:* Improvements in your skin firmness and skin tone

*Exceptional health:* Improved health and well-being, more energy, better mood, and reduced stress

*More strength:* The development of lean muscle, as well as another kind of strength—a boost of confidence

*Blood pressure:* Improved blood pressure from systolic and/or diastolic numbers

In creating *High Fiber Keto*, I used a combination of methods:

1. I collected and distilled information from world-leading researchers and scientists studying how to optimize our metabolism. After I interviewed more than 80 of them in my nine-part docuseries *The Real Skinny on Fat*, I developed High Fiber Keto as an easy-to-follow, metabolism-optimizing diet plan based on scientific research into nutritional ketogenesis and fiber.

2. I scientifically tested the High Fiber Keto diet with a group of women, and the results were incredible. When I saw they had benefits to their bodies, their skin, their minds, and their hormones, I knew this was a program that had metabolism-optimizing powers.

3. I know this program can help you the same way it helped me. I'm a wife, mother, and entrepreneur, and I've felt the effects of a metabolism that was working with major disadvantages, sometimes very profoundly. These experiences

became the foundation of High Fiber Keto and inspired me to find answers. Answers that changed my life. And, I hope, answers that will change yours.

I partnered with researchers at Jacksonville University to conduct a study to test the efficacy of the High Fiber Keto diet. After just three weeks, the study revealed astonishing results.

In the study, 22 women ranging in age from 25 to 60 years old were placed on a ketogenic diet for three weeks to determine how the diet would affect their metabolic, physiological, cognitive, and psychological health. Would they see real changes in such a short period of time?

The answer was a resounding yes!

These study participants spent three weeks on a well-formulated ketogenic diet (WFKD) with a goal of reaching nutritional ketosis by day 21. The women followed a free-living WFKD, meaning they were taught about a ketogenic lifestyle but managed the majority of the diet themselves. They received our sample menus and recipes and were guided toward a diet composed of approximately 50 grams dietary carbohydrates, approximately 20 percent (or 80 to 120 grams) dietary protein, and dietary fat to satiety (approximately 120 to 150 grams). These diets were personalized and the women were free to choose, prepare, and eat foods that fit the diet and their personal preferences.

Before and after the study, researchers measured weight, BMI, waist circumference, waist-to-hip ratio, body composition, blood pressure, circulating markers of metabolic and cardiovascular health, and self-reported mood, anxiety, stress, happiness, and food cravings.

Here are the astonishing results:

91% of the women experienced *weight loss*

91% of the women experienced a *decrease in BMI*

86% of the women *decreased body fat*

95% of women *improved blood pressure*

a) Systolic blood pressure had an average decrease of 9.7 mmHg

b) Diastolic blood pressure had an average change of 4.8 mmHg

73% of women *improved blood glucose*

65% of the women reached *nutritional ketosis* by post testing

Participants reported significant *improvements in anxiety*

Participants reported significant *improvements in food cravings*

Participants reported significant *improvements in skin satisfaction*

This study suggests that carbohydrate restriction can lead to numerous health benefits within three weeks in women. These benefits span overall health improvements, metabolic health, and psychological health and well-being.

It was surprising and exciting to see such encouraging outcomes in just three weeks! I hope these study results will reassure you that you can do it too and be equally successful.

This program offers you everything you need to turn a disadvantage to an advantage. My dream is to walk this journey with you—with each of you. I am offering you a simple, science-backed step-by-step guide for healing your metabolism and enjoying the advantages of metabolic health.

In the pages ahead, you will also find a well-formulated, fiber-rich, nutrient-dense ketogenic diet plan and a movement program that will bring exercise effortlessly into your life. Here's how we'll get there:

*Part I* will take you through the science of the three main components of the High Fiber Keto plan—metabolism, the ketogenic principles and process, and the role of fiber. Learning how they work will give you the biological insights for understanding what it means to put this plan into action. I'll include plenty of quick tips and strategies, and we'll explore all of the additional benefits you can experience when you start High Fiber Keto. (And I have a special WISH list for you in Chapter 4.)

*Part II* is where we'll get into the nuts and bolts of the actions you will take with the High Fiber Keto lifestyle (and yes, I'll tell you which nuts are best)—and how to integrate the specifics into your life. It's absolutely worth acknowledging that keto frightens some people—for a variety of reasons. I, too, had difficulties at first. But I hope that my rundown of how many options you have for foods, nutrients, and simple everyday movement will give you the information and inspiration to try my 22-day plan.

*Part II* is where you'll find the High Fiber Keto plan. This daily plan will give you all you need for a well-formulated, fiber-rich, nutrient-dense ketogenic diet and enable you to use fuel efficiently while nurturing the healthy, vital bacteria in your body. It also includes a movement program that will help you integrate exercise into your life while barely giving it a second thought.

All of the components of High Fiber Keto are designed to optimize your health and give you the metabolic advantage that will allow you to lose weight and keep it off, fix your metabolism so that it works with you and not against you, and restore balance to your hormones so that you not only feel your best, but are better able to mitigate any symptoms associated with major hormonal changes and fluctuations. As the study results show us, carbohydrate restriction can lead to better metabolic and overall health, as well as psychological benefits and improved well-being. A High Fiber Keto diet is an opportunity to experience better health through your commitment to this lifestyle.

Throughout the book you will hear from the women who took part in the High Fiber Keto study. They will share, in their own words, their incredible journeys to metabolism optimization.

*Now* is your moment. Your time to recognize and stand up to what's placing you at a metabolic disadvantage. With the tools that I'm giving you, you can become metabolically flexible. This is your opportunity to turn your dream of being your best self into a reality.

Thank you for allowing me to guide you on this journey.

— Naomi

# PART I

# THE
# SCIENCE
# OF
# HIGH FIBER
# KETO

# CHAPTER ONE

# THE ENGINE
# OF ENERGY

## Understanding How to Optimize Your Metabolism

It doesn't matter if we're talking about fingerprints, DNA, or smiles—you're uniquely *you*. Look at a thousand women, and you'll discover a thousand different shapes, sizes, hormonal compositions, and genetic predispositions that make each one of us unlike any other.

But if you ask the same thousand people what they want out of their bodies, my guess is that many of their answers would come back to the same two words: "More energy."

After all, *energy* is one of those things that we all relate to. We know energy. We feel energy. We crave more energy.

We know how it feels to be strong, vibrant, and resilient in the face of life's challenges. We also know all too well the opposite—how it feels to be drained and to be sluggish, and how we'd rather stay snuggled in bed instead of leaping out of it.

With your health, the energy story doesn't start and stop with what you feel day to day. It actually starts much deeper inside, with how your body generates and uses energy. That process—metabolism—is not only what serves as the power grid for your cells and your body, but it's also what dictates so much of your overall health, including your weight, your body composition, and your ability to manage stress.

Having spent more than two decades in the health and wellness field, I thought I knew all I needed to know about metabolism. And even for those without this experience, I think we all hear *metabolism* and have an idea of what it means. But I initially didn't appreciate its full and powerful effects until I embarked on the journey to better understand my own and that of my mother—to learn how we, and all women, could get healthier and reduce our risk of developing disorders or even metabolic syndrome.

Metabolic syndrome isn't a disease. Instead, it's the name given to a cluster of five risk factors:

- High blood pressure
- High blood sugar
- Excess fat around the waist
- High triglycerides
- Low levels of HDL

By learning about our metabolism, the biology of body composition, and our different fueling systems, we can change the way our bodies look and feel and the way we stay energized and youthful.

Metabolism is a systemic energy system responsible for sustaining life. Every process, every hormone, every heartbeat, and every breath we take is possible only because of our functioning metabolism. While metabolism extends far beyond food, food is still a crucial component because what we eat and drink turns into energy.

During this journey, I have come to think of metabolism as more than just a fat-burning process. I now think of it as *whole-body* metabolism. It includes proper hormone regulation, sleep cycles, the ability to recover, inflammation, optimal immune system, and especially gut health. Whole-body metabolism means having a systemic approach that includes energy but doesn't stop at energy.

Metabolism is the ability for all your systems to work together to ensure the things we value at the top, such as health, energy, and well-being, can be addressed through a systemic approach. With all of the new research that is coming out, we can better understand how our whole body is affected by the system and does not only contribute to your weight or fatigue levels.

Now, here's where it does get a little tricky: all metabolism creates damage in your body; that's the price of doing business. But the problems happen when there's too much damage; overstressing the system is what can lead to disease and health problems. That's where an optimized metabolism comes in. The more efficient it is, the better you will be at managing it—and the more resilient you will become.

One way to think about metabolism is as your body's master puppeteer of the different mechanisms that influence weight and fat storage, cellular systems, immune function, hormonal makeup, and microbiome. It might seem that this puppeteer works independently, pulling and yanking at your body's systems in whatever way it darn well pleases, but it doesn't.

Here's the thing that has become so clear to me: *You* are in control of the fuel that feeds your metabolism to have a positive effect on your weight, your energy, your ability to fend off disease, and to keep your body healthy and functioning as efficiently as possible. Now, to be clear, there are some genetic factors that are beyond your control (PCOS or endometriosis, for example), but things like diet, exercise, and stress management are within your control. This is the important take-home.

*You* get to direct the systems of your body. *You* have input on how your body burns or stores fat. *You* have input on your own energy levels by managing your cellular energy processes. *You* get to be the puppeteer of the puppeteer.

This change in the way you think about metabolism—a metabolism makeover—will help you change the way your body works, as well as how your body feels. In this chapter, I want to take you inside this miraculous and majestic system. When you understand the most important elements of how energy works, you will see how High Fiber Keto is really the key for improving your body's engine.

Your mission? To optimize your metabolism.

# METABOLISM OPTIMIZER ONE

## First Fuel: Fat

We all know that food serves as fuel for the body, so the best way to think about metabolism is as the engine. It's what determines how well your whole body runs.

While many individual factors determine your metabolic rate (that is, the amount of daily energy needed to support all your life functions and activities), we should start by thinking about metabolism in ideal terms. What would the dream metabolic engine look like?

In technical terms, your dream engine would use all its energy sources as efficiently as possible, finding balance for your own body and learning not to rely on the short-lived fuel source of glucose. Instead, it would turn to your body's largest fuel source—fat—for primary energy to power your immune, cardiovascular, and neurological system. This dream metabolic engine would make your body run like an electric car: efficiently, powerfully, and emitting very few waste products.

Driving would put little stress on your engine and other critical parts, so the body of a car would experience minimal damage—even with the wear and tear of driving. Additionally, your vehicle could function at a high level all day long and be charged (refueled) at longer intervals. Finally, you would get your energy from the rechargeable batteries inside of yourself, and thus your energy supply would come from within—it would just need to be supported.

Unfortunately, most of us don't have a metabolism like an electric car. Instead, the typical person functions more like a 10-year-old, gas-powered vehicle: inefficient and emitting lots of metabolic waste products. The people at a true metabolic disadvantage? They're more like big trucks, putting out tons of exhaust and using a lot of energy (and thus needing to be constantly refueled). Over time, these metabolic wastes in the body can start to impair the function of our vital organs and ultimately compromise our health.[1]

But regardless of how efficiently we're operating, in reality our bodies are most like hybrid vehicles, which have two distinct energy sources: the internal combustion engine and an electric generator.

Similarly, we have two primary sources of energy to fuel our bodies: glucose and fat.

Glucose is indeed a fuel that can be used to move our bodies quickly for brief periods of time, and it has an intended role—to fuel the brain, red blood cells, and sometimes skeletal muscle—but the energy doesn't last. Most people start to feel hungry, fatigued, unfocused, or all of the above.

So the goal is to be more like the electric car and run off your body's largest and longest-lasting energy depot of fat and ketones all day long, rather than the glucose (which gets used or stored quickly), with as little waste as possible. It is important to note that glucose is an important fuel for the body. It is the primary fuel for the major organs, such as the brain and red blood cells, and one our muscles use for quick, powerful bursts of energy. The issue is that we often consume more than our body typically needs.

Now, you may wonder why the goal isn't to be a Ferrari, with its super-fast and super-powerful engine. The problem is that there's a price for that speed: you burn through fuel too quickly and constantly have to refuel, as well as put a lot of wear and tear on the car. This is what happens when your body runs exclusively on glucose as an energy source: you may get brief periods of speed and power, but you are constantly looking to refuel—and you end up burning out all of your key components over time.

## METABOLISM OPTIMIZER TWO

### Muscle Mass/Body Fat

For so long, we have used "weight" as a proxy for our health. And while weight can be an important number to give you an indication of how healthy you are or aren't, it's really not the best number . . . or the only number. Why? Because it doesn't take into consideration that ratio of lean muscle mass to body fat.

For an optimized metabolism, you want to start thinking less about weight in pounds, but more so about your total body composition. It's one of the best indicators to give you insight into how your body is functioning, it helps identify health and risk factors, and it's an essential tool to help let you know if you are at risk for metabolically driven diseases. Plus, it's a much more scientifically sound measure.

Body composition is your ratio of fat to fat-free mass (muscle mass, bones, and water) in the body. Body fat is an essential tissue responsible for protecting our vital organs, temperature regulation, hormone balance, and gut health. Too little or too much body fat can lead to direct disruptions in metabolic health. Recently, research has shown the location of this body fat has a substantial effect on your health. For example, higher fat around your midsection is closely tied to metabolic and cardiac health. Higher body fat in the midsection is dangerous because of its proximity to our major metabolic organs, including the liver and gut. It has the direct ability to disrupt our metabolic processes and over time leads to chronically higher risk for diabetes mellitus, stroke, and cardiac events.[2]

Body composition is also directly tied to metabolic rate, or the amount of energy it takes to fuel all major functions in your body. Higher levels of skeletal muscle and lower levels of body fat can lead to a higher metabolic rate.[3]

Metabolic rate—the amount of energy your body needs to sustain life—can fluctuate, depending on things like your body comp, activity level, stress levels, and reproductive stage. The goal is to find balance in your metabolic rate and use fuel most efficiently.

As we age, our metabolic rate naturally begins to slow down, which matches the slow decline in muscle mass and steady increase in body fat that we accumulate.[4] Diet and exercise influence our body fat and amount of skeletal muscle, though skeletal muscle is more metabolically active than fat. And that's a good thing, as our bodies are always in flux, and it is common to have varying levels of fat and skeletal muscle throughout the years.

Because muscle is more metabolically active, it requires more calories to sustain itself than fat.[5] Skeletal muscle is metabolically active because it is in a constant state of remodeling. Muscle takes an enormous amount of energy to build, recover, and maintain. Body fat requires very little energy to sustain itself. A simple way to think about it is this: The more fat you have, the less fuel you burn. The more lean mass you have, the more fuel you burn.

That's why body composition (or "body comp")—and a healthy amount of fat—is so vital to your overall metabolic rate.

That then begs the question: What is the right amount of fat? After all, most of us know that there are clear dangers with having too much fat. And having too little fat can disrupt health. Hormonal function, bone health, healthy skin and hair, and sleep can all be negatively affected when body fat is too low.

For most women a healthy body-fat ratio ranges from approximately 20 to 30 percent. Now, the challenge with that number is that it's not easy to quickly assess (in the way you can read a scale, for example). There are body-comp scales and expensive ways to have professionals measure it more accurately than an at-home scales but these are not necessarily easily accessible to everyone.

While body composition is currently the gold standard for estimating lean tissue to fat mass, these measurements may be difficult to assess, track over time, and at times, interpret. So although they may not give exact numbers, it is important to find accessible methods to better understand your body's health without having to undergo a body composition analysis.

Then the question becomes: How do you assess where you are? What data should you use to see how you're doing? Let's look at a few of the markers that aren't technically considered body comp (in terms of measuring actual tissue) but are manageable ways to get a sense of where you are.

> *BMI (body mass index):* BMI is a clinical tool used to determine your ratio of height to weight (not body composition or actual tissue). Using various BMI calculators online, you can enter your weight in pounds and height. "Normal" BMI ranges between 18.4 and 24.9, but this number only considers height and weight. And while BMI is easily accessible, it is one dimensional with a lot of room for inaccuracy and does not account for type or quality of tissue.

Typically, we hear of risks associated with high BMI, but a low BMI is not a guarantee that your body fat is in the healthy range. Recent studies have shown that individuals can have a low BMI but a high body-fat percentage. Even more concerning, these individuals are at increased risk of mortality. And if you have a lot of lean muscle, it may cause a higher BMI, even if you have less body fat. BMI can be helpful but, in many cases, it is misleading, inaccurate, and difficult to interpret.

More and more research is moving away from BMI standards for women's health and instead turning to more focused styles of measurement.

> *Waist Circumference:* Recent research has suggested that waist circumference is one of the most powerful clinical tools a woman can use to better understand her metabolic health.[6] There are times we may be making progress but where the scale may not reflect it. Waist circumference is now being found to be a better predictor or indicator of metabolic health.[7] It still has its limitations but more clinical studies are finding that increases in belly fat are integrated with overall metabolic health. Waist circumference is something any of us can track on our own but knowing how to interpret it is key. This measurement backs us away from the scale and allows us to focus less on overall weight and more on the type of weight that directly and indirectly affects our health.

It is important to note this number fluctuates just like all parts of our bodies do, so while we want to bring it within optimal range, as long as your body is trending in the right direction, improvements are being made. Currently, World Health Organization standards for waist circumference are less than 35 inches (88 cm) for women.[8] However, waist circumference is affected by age and race. Although there are ranges to consider, these ranges are being further investigated to ensure a broader representation.

Carbohydrate restriction has consistently shown improvements in both body composition and waist circumference. It varies from woman to woman but reducing sugars and increasing healthier fat, whole-food options seem to consistently show better weight management and decreased waist circumference measurements.[9,10]

*Waist-to-Hip Ratio:* Waist-to-hip ratio is an equally powerful tool for better insight into metabolic health.[11] Recent research suggests it may even be more specific to cardiometabolic health than waist circumference or BMI.[12] Waist-to-hip ratio is also tied to long-term health. For example, one study found it may help predict 10-year cardiovascular risk.[13] But, like waist circumference, it must be correctly interpreted and taken as part of the whole picture, not just one piece.

Wrap a tape measure around the smallest part of your waist, and then measure your hips at the widest part. Divide the waist by the hip. You want a ratio that is under 0.85, according to guidelines from the Word Health Organization.[14] This is a good indicator to see where fat is sitting; more fat around the waist means you're at a higher metabolic risk.

Research shows that where you hold excess body fat may be closely tied to cardiac, hormonal, and metabolic health. Visceral fat, or the fat found around the organs in the abdominal area, is needed for cushioning and hormonal control. When this type of fat increases, it is in extremely close proximity to major metabolic organs such as the liver and gut. Visceral fat may leak into circulation and be sent to the liver for processing, adding an unexpected additional load for the liver to manage. This in turn can cause major disruptions in the system and over time can lead to increased risk for developing the primary metabolic disorders that affect women's heath, including cardiometabolic diseases, type 2 diabetes, and strokes.

*Subjective Observations:* Changes in your body can't always be seen or aren't always measured, but don't be afraid to put some stock in questions (and answers) that include subjective data. How do you feel? How do your clothes fit? Do you feel less bloated? Think about these things throughout the day, such as before and after meals, when you wake up, and before you go to sleep. These less objective observations can clue you in about your progress. And they can often mean much more than the number you read on the scale. Don't minimize the impact of these kinds of markers.

To be clear, the goal here isn't about appearance or athletic performance. The goal is to strike the right body-comp balance so that you help build an efficient and effective metabolism—one that supports lean tissue and doesn't slow down because of a higher percentage of body fat.

## METABOLISM OPTIMIZER THREE

### Ketones: The Fourth Macronutrient

Before the electric car, most people thought that gasoline was the only fuel source for cars. Although it is recognized that some types of gasoline are higher quality than others, it has now become widely accepted that cars can run more efficiently and emit fewer toxins with another fuel source—electricity. Similarly, it's only been within the past couple decades that ketones, which are more efficient at producing energy and produce less metabolic waste than glucose, have been discovered as the body's super fuel source.

Ketones are produced as a by-product of fat metabolism anytime the body is burning a lot of fat. This can happen when you are fasting or on the High Fiber Keto diet. When glucose from carbs is in short supply, your body breaks down fat into fatty acids and glycerol. These can be used to fuel many of your cells but cannot be used by your brain cells because fatty acids and glycerol convert into energy too slowly for your brain's rapid energy need.

At this point, your liver steps in and converts the fatty acids and glycerol into sugars and ketones. Your liver sends these ketones into your bloodstream to be used as fuel for your brain, muscles, and other organs such as the heart. This burning of ketones for fuel is called *nutritional ketosis*.

Nutritional ketosis is your best and most efficient means of fueling your cells, which is why a ketogenic diet is so important to the metabolism story: your fuel choice determines the efficiency and longevity of the engine.

I will share more with you about the importance of nutritional ketosis in Chapter 2 but this discussion lays the groundwork for a deeper understanding of the ketogenic process.

# METABOLISM OPTIMIZER FOUR

## Metabolism: Energy Efficiency

From a weight management standpoint, the faster your metabolism, the more calories you burn 24/7. That may seem like a fat-burner's dream, but that's not necessarily the case. Being at either end of the speed spectrum is not ideal.

> *The problem with slow:* The main problem with a puttering metabolism: it puts you at risk for metabolically related conditions, increases in body fat, and decreases in muscle mass. A big reason why so many people have trouble maintaining weight loss through extreme calorie-restricted diets is that their metabolism slows down due to the lack of incoming fuel. The body preserves the fuel it does have when none is coming in. Ultimately, this creates a cycle of slowing metabolism, which contributes to weight gain.

> *The problem with fast:* While slow metabolism is certainly a problem, that doesn't mean you want the exact opposite. A rocket-fast metabolism has its downsides, too. Stephen Anton, Ph.D., a professor and chief of clinical research at the University of Florida's Institute on Aging, is an expert on metabolic health. He has devoted his career to studying how a person's lifestyle can either improve their health or increase their risk for obesity, cardiovascular disease, and metabolic disease conditions.

He shared that your metabolism can technically be both your friend and your foe. You see, the process of creating energy (your metabolism) also produces reactive oxygen species (ROS) and free radicals that can damage cells, trigger inflammation, cause oxidative stress, and accelerate aging. The faster your metabolism runs, the more ROS it produces, which is why many experts now believe that a slower metabolism may be the key to living longer because it creates less metabolic stress on your body.

This makes sense. If you put your foot all the way down on the gas pedal every time you drive a car, you'll damage the engine. Too fast can be as damaging as too slow.

> *The Bio-Optimized Metabolism:* Ideally, you want a stable metabolism that works efficiently. That's a bio-optimized metabolism—one that doesn't run too slow (which makes you more susceptible to weight gain) or too fast (so it doesn't produce higher levels of ROS and lead to inflammation). In other words, instead of looking at your metabolism as something you always need to shift into a different gear, it's about finding a middle ground that checks every box in terms of wellness. This is what my 22-day plan does as it nudges your metabolism, through food and movement, into this sweet spot of energy efficiency.

## METABOLISM OPTIMIZER FIVE

### Outsmart Age and Genetics

Though it's true that many people experience a slower metabolic rate as they age, it's not entirely clear how much of this decline is caused by the aging process versus unhealthy lifestyle changes that we make as we get older. One factor: Many people don't exercise as much as they did when they were younger, and this lack of activity can lead to a loss of lean muscle (which then contributes to a slower metabolism). Muscle mass and fat both carry hormones, so if your body comp is off, you risk disrupting your hormone balance—that is, if your muscle mass is too low, you might not get enough or if your level of fat is too high, you may get too much of a hormone you need.

Our body composition changes slowly at first, and we may or may not notice that we are carrying less muscle and more fat. But over time this process accelerates and can leave most women wondering what happened to the body they had in their 20s and 30s. Women are at particular risk because after menopause, we no longer have as much estrogen to help us burn body fat.

As you have learned, the less lean muscle you have, the slower your metabolism runs because that lean mass burns more fuel. Regular exercise and eating the right foods can help minimize or prevent that loss.[15]

In addition, it's difficult to separate the interaction between changes that typically occur during aging and a person's lifestyle. For example, do more responsibilities mean less attention to healthy habits? Do older people stop doing certain things (vigorous exercise) because they think they're too old?

The point: While aging does mean there are some inevitable slowdowns in various biological processes, it's not the definitive destiny that you might assume. Controlling your metabolism through various lifestyle techniques can, well, slow down a slowdown.

Speaking of speed, you're probably thinking about individuals who may appear to be able to eat whatever they want without gaining weight (or the opposite). While some people believe that they're saddled with a slow metabolism due to their genes, Dr. Anton explained that the vast majority of us do not suffer from a genetically caused extremely low metabolic rate. In fact, less than 3 percent of the population experience true genetically caused obesity.[16]

That said, genetics does have *some* influence over your metabolism. But to what degree has been debated for some time. In fact, Catherine Saenz, Ph.D., R.D., CSCS, at Jacksonville University, shared with me this insight: If you looked at the resting metabolisms of hundreds of individuals they may—for the most part—sit within a specific window, since the majority of the energy we require is used to fuel our body's basic functioning while at rest to keep us alive. But two factors that we do know affect your metabolism are (1) the types of foods you are eating and (2) how much and what type of activity you're doing at that moment.

The point: Genetics has some influence over metabolic rate, but you do have some control over metabolic rate as well.

# METABOLISM OPTIMIZER SIX

## Increase Your Cell Power

In your body, you don't have a metabolism organ. Instead, all organs and systems in the body are involved in metabolism. Our organs are working 24 hours a day to ensure we can sustain our life and each one functions at a different metabolic rate. In fact, our most metabolically active organs are the ones we may not even consider to be part of the process, including the heart, liver, brain, and kidneys.[17] In order for this system to occur seamlessly, metabolism must begin at the cellular level all throughout your body, where every cell goes through the process of creating energy and removing waste, producing energy for our organs and whole body.

The generators? They're called *mitochondria*, the structures in your cells that are the source of more than 90 percent of your body's energy. To produce this power, your mitochondria require oxygen from the air you breathe and fat and glucose from the food you eat.

So while the process happens at a microscopic level and you can't see results the way you would see, say, a toned arm that you work out, you can have an effect on your mitochondria. And when you improve their function, they enhance the energy-generating levels in your body.

These are some ways to improve mitochondria and metabolic functions:

> *Diet:* Whenever mitochondria oxidize a macronutrient—whether carbohydrates, proteins, fats, or ketones—what's left behind are unstable free radicals that can damage DNA, cells, and protein. But when you metabolize ketones for energy instead of glucose, something magical happens in the body: The mitochondrial function improves and starts producing higher amounts of ATP (the energy currency of the cell) more efficiently while leaving fewer free radicals behind. Ketones are super fuel, so when you fuel your engine this way, you produce energy more efficiently while simultaneously creating less damage to your cells, particularly your mitochondria.[18]

*Sleep:* It's important to get five sleep cycles or somewhere between seven and nine hours of high-quality sleep every night. When you sleep, your body goes through the very natural process of switching your energy source from glucose to fatty acids and fatty-acid derived ketones—and our bodies repair and regenerate the vital tissues and organs. Sleep is so important for our metabolic health because when we sleep, we are clearing out waste products and restoring our hormonal levels to function optimally. Many studies have shown that there are sleep-specific metabolic changes, including reductions in body temperature[19] and energy expenditure and increases in growth hormone that work to restore our metabolic health.[20] If sleep is disturbed or insufficient, unhealthy metabolic states, such as insulin resistance, inflammation, and obesity, can develop.[21] Tip: It's best to get some sleep before 11 P.M., because that's when the most restorative cycles tend to occur.

*Reducing Stress:* Engage in some activity that is relaxing to the mind-body, such as meditation, listening to music, or taking a warm bath. Chronic stress can adversely affect metabolism because it leads to elevated levels of the stress hormone cortisol, which taps into your energy stores, including stored forms of glucose and fat and your precious muscle for energy. According to Dr. Anton, although stress reactions burn calories initially, chronic stress can lead to a reduction in metabolism in the long run due to the loss of muscle that occurs when cortisol is constantly elevated. Additionally, cortisol can also stimulate appetite and lead to overconsumption of foods that are high in sugar and fat. If cortisol remains high, these unhealthy eating patterns and use of muscle protein for energy can ultimately lead to insulin resistance, which we know puts us at a metabolic disadvantage.

*Exercise:* When you work out, you are giving your body a tune-up so that it can more efficiently use its super fuel. The effect seems to be acute and lasts 24 to 72 hours, depending on the intensity of the exercise. This is because exercise, particularly high-intensity interval training and weight training, enhances the muscles' uptake of glucose, which reduces it in the bloodstream. By exercising first thing in the morning, you not only burn more calories, you increase your metabolic rate throughout the day and train your body to run off fat and ketones for energy. (Note: If you can't exercise in the morning, don't be hard on yourself; it's best to find a time that you will exercise consistently rather than not exercise at all.)

*Move throughout the Day:* Just regular movement can help your body utilize glucose for energy and also help combat the post-meal rise in insulin and glucose levels. Take a stroll after a meal since it both helps your body digest the food and also helps clear glucose from the bloodstream. A study published in 2013 in the journal *Diabetes Care* found that in prediabetic, older adults, three short walks each day after meals were as effective at reducing blood sugar over 24 hours as a single 45-minute walk. Even more important, taking a walk in the evening substantially lowered blood sugar levels in these same participants compared with not walking.

In addition, other smaller tactics that have been shown to help improve mitochondrial function include ingestion of mitochondrial nutrients (like vitamin B), exposure to sunlight, and cold and heat exposure (which triggers the body to make metabolic shifts to adjust to the changing temperatures).

### Discover Your Metabolism's True Age

So, are *you* at a metabolic disadvantage? And is it holding you back from experiencing your best weight, energy, and health? Dr. Anton and I created an assessment that reveals the true age of your metabolism and the simple quick switches you can do right away to begin gaining an optimized metabolism. Go to NaomiWhittel/metabolism.com and use the code *high fiber keto* to get your results. But remember, no matter what the numbers may say about your metabolism, changing them to work for you instead of against you is what *High Fiber Keto* is all about.

These six optimizers are designed to strengthen and power your metabolic processes and avoid metabolic syndrome. Studies show that people with metabolic syndrome have a five times higher risk of mortality compared with those who don't have this syndrome.[22]

This table is an easy reference to help you measure your current metabolic health based on the five risk factors[23] you learned about earlier:

| Factor | Risk Factor | Effect |
|---|---|---|
| Blood pressure | Greater than 130/85 | Anything above this magic number doesn't just put you at risk for heart disease; it can cause brain health issues, kidney damage, eyesight problems, nerve damage, and even bone loss. |
| Blood sugar | Above 100 mg/dL | When it stays too high for too long, it can trigger a series of issues ranging from skin problems, kidney and nerve damage to heart disease and diabetes. |
| Abdominal fat | 35 inches or higher for women (38 for men) | This can nearly double your risk of dying prematurely and makes you more likely to experience a wide variety of health issues, including cancer, heart disease, and even dementia. |
| Triglyceride levels | Higher than 150 mg/dL | Triglycerides (found in your blood) are the most common form of fat in your body; anything higher than this number is strongly associated with significant lipid abnormalities, insulin resistance, and cardiovascular disease. |
| HDL (good) cholesterol | Less than 50 mg/dL in women (40 mg/dL in men) | High-density lipoprotein (HDL) helps bring excess cholesterol in your blood back to your liver where it can be broken down and removed from your body. |

Now, according to Dr. Anton, we also should be aware of the unofficial sixth factor: chronic, low-grade inflammation. Many experts consider it to be an indicator of metabolic syndrome because of the growing amount of evidence linking it to disease.

At first glance, inflammation can be a good thing,[24] as long as it is temporary. Inflammation is part of the body's natural defense mechanism, signaling the immune system to remove harmful stimuli and begin the healing process. Generally, there are two types of inflammation, acute and chronic. Acute inflammation occurs as an immediate response to trauma with a relatively short duration (lasting from minutes to days).

Chronic inflammation, however, begins with a cellular response but stays active regardless of any immediate threat to the body and can last for months or even years. Eventually, if the inflammatory response continues unabated, the immune system begins to attack healthy tissue and organs, which can impair the body's function and lead to a host of health[25] conditions.

We now know that chronic inflammation, even at a low level, contributes to many life-threatening conditions, including auto-immune disorders,[26] heart disease,[27] Alzheimer's,[28] psychiatric disease,[29] and cancer,[30] among others. Moreover, there is now evidence that chronic inflammation may contribute to early death, making it a true public health issue.[31] We do know that levels of inflammation tend to be higher in individuals who are at a metabolic disadvantage and have one or more of the five indicators of metabolic syndrome. Although the link between inflammation and metabolic syndrome is not fully understood, some believe the connection may be that adipose tissue releases increased amounts of adipokines (inflammatory cytokines, proteins that influence the immune system), while others believe insulin resistance is responsible for causing more inflammatory cytokines to circulate[32] in the body.

What *is* known is that when you eat a diet high in sugar, your immune system reacts as if it's fighting off an infection. In fact, just having a single can of soda has been shown to increase inflammatory markers in the blood.[33] That's why becoming a fat burner—in addition to reducing your body fat through a ketogenic diet and more movement—can lower some of that unnecessary, all-day inflammation.

Although it is possible to have only one of the five official metabolic risk factors (six if you include chronic inflammation), these factors frequently co-occur. And having three or more is all it takes to be diagnosed with metabolic syndrome. Of course, the more risk factors you have, the greater your risk of heart disease, stroke, diabetes, and other health problems. But what scares many experts I spoke with is that most of these metabolic risk factors have no easy-to-spot signs or symptoms, with the exception of measuring your waistline.

In essence, this is what has driven me to create *High Fiber Keto*—my desire to give you the road map so you can reduce or eliminate these risk factors and go from being at a metabolic disadvantage to having an optimized metabolism.

This ideal metabolic state happens when you are using energy efficiently (remember, not too fast and not too slow). And it looks like this:

- You're improving your body composition by losing fat and increasing lean muscle, which means a healthier appearance and, more importantly, a healthier metabolic system.

- You're focused, energized, and satiated after meals.

- You're using your own fat efficiently and as intended, as your primary source of energy, while optimizing the health of your organs, muscles, and mitochondria.

- You're preserving glucose for its necessary roles and relying on fat, the largest energy depot in the body for fuel.

How do you get an optimized metabolism? It starts with the subject of Chapter 2, learning how to use and maximize your body's most preferred fuel source: ketones.

# DEBRA

## *I feel like I got my life back.*

I have to be honest: I went into High Fiber Keto with some anxiety. I've tried so many plans over the years and just have struggled to maintain any success. But then I gave it a try, and after the first week? I was in it. Why? The scale was a huge motivator, yes, and I just *felt* better.

Before this, my energy had been spiraling downward for years. I always felt tired, and I never wanted to take on anything extra. *Overwhelmed* is the word I kept coming back to.

High Fiber Keto helped me learn about the power of the food we consume and about how it could make the difference between feeling tired and feeling energized. And in the end, that was really the difference between wearing my husband's T-shirts and being comfortable in my own clothes, the difference between battling skin inflammation and glowing skin, and the difference between feeling like I was in a constant fog to wanting to live life.

I haven't felt this good in years, and I am post-menopausal! My husband got his wife back, and I feel like I got my life back.

# CHAPTER TWO

# THE
# KETO CURE

## How and Why Optimal Nutrition Can Drive Your Metabolic State

I fell in love with keto and enjoyed the benefits of high fat before I even knew what keto was. When I was growing up in England, my mother made sure that everything I ate was healthy and consisted of whole foods, so I started every day with whole-food sources of fats. I ate spoonfuls of cod liver oil, as well as whole butter, full-fat cream, and a variety of cheeses for breakfast.

But when I was a teenager and living in the U.S., I decided I wanted to eat like my friends. So I started every morning the way they did—with toast or a bowl of cereal. I didn't know it at the time, of course, but I was getting a big lesson in how crucial nutrition is to how we fuel our bodies.

When I ate the way that my family taught me to eat, I felt good. I had energy and an overall positive attitude. But when I transitioned into more simple carbohydrates, more processed foods, and more junk, it set the stage for me to slowly become more and more dependent on sugar—something that affected my sleep patterns, my thought processes, and my health.

And this was key to understanding the whole metabolic state. There are so many things that influence metabolism, including weight, blood pressure, insulin sensitivity, blood sugar, hormones, sleep, and stress. All of these things can cause metabolic dysfunction, leading to cardiovascular disease, diabetes, GI dysfunction, mental health problems, and other potential life-threatening conditions.

While it's true that metabolic health is affected by some things you can't change (age and genetics), the fact is that much of it is controllable through choices, through lifestyle, and through decisions we make every day. And that's why in the last few months of 2017 I turned to a keto lifestyle and I have been going strong ever since. I wanted to take control of the things I could control—the number one thing being what I ate.

Even with my access to experts, I discovered that either the answers aren't easily available, or at times we're not even asking the right questions. And that means there are a whole lot of people who are "keto confused." If you're like many people who were brought up on lasagna, pizza, and buckets of fries, it can be challenging to wrap your head around what keto means and how to make it your new way of eating.

This chapter is about helping you learn about and navigate the keto lifestyle—to see how it works and better understand it. You probably fall into one of these three categories:

- *The Keto Curious:* Those who know about ketogenic diets but have never tried one because they seem too complex to understand, feel too limiting in terms of diet, or appear too difficult to adhere to.

- *The Keto Crushed:* Those who have tried a ketogenic diet, but found it either a struggle or too much of a sacrifice.

- *The Keto Confident:* Those who presently enjoy a keto lifestyle and may be experiencing *some* of the benefits that can come from utilizing ketones—but with awareness and background, could start to explore more areas ketones may affect.

# WHAT IS KETO?

You probably have a good idea about the purpose of food: it's what provides us with available energy for our body's systems. Whatever your body doesn't use? That gets stored. The key hormone in this process is insulin, because it carries glucose directly to cells that need energy. Anything not used immediately gets distributed to a few places—some into blood glucose, some into muscle, and the rest converted to fat, a form of stored energy. Fat can distribute that energy to many vital organs or when you're not getting consistent energy (when you're sleeping or exercising, for example).

This system works really well. Your body has an innate sense of what it needs to do and what it wants to do to run smoothly.

But the system starts to malfunction when we consume foods high in sugar. This triggers insulin, and when insulin goes up, fat metabolism slows. And that's a problem because the body becomes insulin resistant (you need more glucose to trigger the system), and the body becomes less efficient at using fat, instead turning to glucose as energy.

The effect: You increase your fat, but you don't utilize it as well, which means you increase your fat storage. And that throws *everything* off. Hormones. Energy. Inflammation is triggered. Your organs are stressed.

And that's where keto comes in.

The keto diet reduces insulin-spiking foods, including high-glycemic foods or high-carb foods, such as starches, breads, and pasta.

To accomplish the goal of managing insulin, you have to manage carbs. Natural intuition sometimes pushes us to replace carbohydrates with protein rather than fat. Protein is an essential nutrient but its role is structural; it is not an ideal energy source for the body. In fact, the body tries hard to not turn to protein for energy at all. Additionally, some amino acids in protein are glucogenic, meaning they are able to help synthesize glucose and end up triggering the insulin response you are trying to manage. This approach can leave you feeling foggy-brained, tired, and with GI discomfort. If you reduce your carbohydrate intake, especially to about 50 grams per day, the ideal place to start in a ketogenic diet, you'll be switching your main fuel from dietary carbohydrate to dietary fat. Fat is our most energy-dense macronutrient and can be found in plenty of whole foods. It's the preferred fuel source for many of our major organs. The goal is to retrain our bodies how to turn it into our primary fuel source.

That's what the keto diet is: a way of eating that is low carb, moderate protein, and high fat that gets your body using fuel efficiently. With this macronutrient breakdown, your body turns to fat (and its by-product, ketones) as its primary source of fuel—both from your own fat stores and the fat sources you eat. This is in addition to small amounts of glucose, the readily available energy source that's quickly pumped into the bloodstream with carbohydrates. By maintaining suggested levels of dietary protein, you are really focusing on flipping your carb and fat portions. If you do this continuously for a few days, you will reach a state called *nutritional ketosis*.

There are two primary ways to reach nutritional ketosis:

- extreme calorie reduction
- maintaining calories but drastically reducing your dietary carbohydrate intake while simultaneously maintaining your dietary protein consumption and increasing your dietary fat intake

Nutritional ketosis is a state where your body is burning through such high levels of fat that it produces additional metabolic by-products called *ketones*. Ketones are actually typical by-products whenever we use fat, so they are always in circulation. However, since fat is not usually our primary source of energy, the levels we have circulating are much much lower. When we increase our fat intake and decrease our carbohydrate level to the point of switching over to relying more heavily on fat, our bodies make ketones in higher quantities.

These levels are all within normal physiological range, or levels very well tolerated in the body. Nutritional ketosis is typically within the ranges of 0.5 to 5.0 mmol/L and is the state where many people report increases in energy, increases in mental clarity, decreased GI distress, more focus, improvements in mood, and improvements in body composition. Once you remove your reliance on carbohydrates, you also remove the constant highs and lows that come with fluctuating blood sugar levels. The goal of a keto diet is to maintain blood sugar throughout the day, supply a steady state of energy through fat we eat or have, and become more efficient at how we use fuel and manage it from a whole-body standpoint—from our brain to our heart to our mind.

## THE SCIENCE OF KETO: DON'T FEAR FAT

It's not uncommon for people to hear the word "fat," and think it's a bad thing, since too much body fat can be. But when people hear the word *fat* when it comes to the macronutrient, they tend to think the same thing: fat in the body is bad, so fat in food must be too. But this way of thinking extends far beyond just the word itself. It started because of the way we have thought about diet as research developed and because of the way that fat has been portrayed as a dietary villain.

Anti-fat discussions started in the 1950s, back when lipoproteins—particularly low-density lipoprotein (LDL) and high-density lipoprotein (HDL)—were discovered in blood by Ancel Keys. It became common for researchers to explore force-feeding animals both saturated fat and cholesterol to see their effect on heart disease. But the fallout from all that fat fear caused omega-3 fatty acids, monounsaturated fat, polyunsaturated fat, and saturated fat—to be lumped in with the bad-for-you fats such as trans fats and partially hydrogenated oils. And suddenly, all types of fat were a foe.

What has the result of this research and eventual diet dogma led to? It is now commonly accepted that eating fat will make you "fat," despite compelling evidence suggesting otherwise, and that high-quality carbohydrates are both the bulk and preferred manner of eating for most people. These precepts have been around for decades, with research connecting increases in fat in the diet with increased risk of atherosclerosis and cardiovascular disease discounting what we now understand about nutrient-dense whole foods, inflammation, hormones, and monounsaturated and omega-3 fats.

Because of this mind-set, we've been programmed to feel that fat is the enemy. And since that time, it's led many to follow a low-fat, high-carb diet and to toss aside or minimize foods naturally rich in fat such as olive, coconut, or avocado oils and avocados, dairy, and animal proteins.

When the first dietary guidelines were created to help combat heart disease as it rose in the 1980s, they encouraged less dietary fat and more carbohydrates.[1] Americans carefully and obediently heeded the advice to reduce fat intake and increase whole grains, starchy carbohydrates, and plentiful fruits. The consumption of carbohydrates rose—as did the fear of fat.

As people have taken that nutritional advice, our collective health has been made worse for it. Researchers in the United States went back to see how health outcomes have fared after the changes in recommendations in dietary approaches. When looking more deeply into how these health outcomes have matched these changes in diet, health deteriorations coincided with when we started eating higher amounts of refined carbs and fewer fats. Obesity and diabetes in this country continue to rise to epidemic numbers. For the vast majority, a blanket suggestion to follow high-carb and low-fat diets has not been working, and it's causing people to struggle and suffer health-wise. The shift to moderate- to high-carb diets (and reducing emphasis on fat) goes against basic biology and scientific evidence about how we should fuel our bodies.

**How we fuel our bodies:** Your body relies on glucose (sugar) and fat as its two primary fuel sources. Because the traditional Western diet is carb-centric (deriving roughly 45 to 65 percent of its calories from carbohydrates), most people are what experts call "sugar burners," or those who rely primarily on glucose for energy.

The majority of glucose needs can be produced by the liver at 130 to 160 grams per day, but we tend to consume that or more in just one meal. Instead, our goal should be to reduce our reliance on this common, short-lived fuel source and turn on our body's natural fuel sources.

Our body stores a very small amount of carbohydrates, enough for only a few miles of activity. There are several ways to replenish this energy store, but the most common way is to consume foods rich in carbohydrates. The more we turn to external sources of energy, the less our body uses its already existing internal sources of energy. This is especially true for body fat. The higher the carb content in the diet, the more the body relies on carbs and less on fat for energy, meaning that the body turns to fat only a fraction of what it should or could. And when the metabolic switch never gets flipped, during the times when we should be able to access our fat stores, our body will insist on turning to (or asking for) carbohydrate sources.

**The effect of a carb-heavy diet:** Consuming high levels of carbs and fats together can lead to a host of cardiovascular and metabolic and obesity-related disorders such as type 2 diabetes, hypertension, and heart disease. Unhealthy metabolic states can typically increase hunger levels, which can promote weight and fat gain, which can promote higher hunger levels, which can promote weight gain, and on and on. The balance between dietary carbohydrate and dietary fat is very delicate. If carbohydrates are not decreased enough and the diet is increased in fat, it too can lead to major health issues. In order for our body to turn to fat for fuel, carbohydrates have to be reduced to adequate and individualized levels.

It should be said that some people can handle dietary carbs (especially if they are from whole-food sources) very well. But for the majority of us—especially when faced with increased stress, aging, or more sedentary lifestyles—it is not the best type of energy to use. We do much better with a lower-carb diet that emphasizes whole, high-quality foods rich in natural fats, high-quality proteins, and limited but nutrient-dense sources of carbs.

**What happens with carbs:** Every time you eat carbs, they are digested into simple sugars and absorbed into your bloodstream, causing your blood sugar levels to rise. Your body wants to maintain a very narrow range of circulating sugar in your bloodstream; 70 to 99 mg/dL (about a teaspoon) is considered normal under fasting conditions, according to Brittanie Volk, Ph.D., R.D.

Blood sugars respond to all carbohydrates, including fruits and veggies, and to a lesser extent, animal proteins. Depending on what you eat, your blood sugar can rise dramatically. In response to a surge of sugar, your pancreas will release a substantial amount of insulin, a hormone that helps remove sugar from your blood and place it into your cells where it can be used for energy—or stored as unwanted body fat. But what's worse is that over time—especially if you're a sugar burner—your cells will become less responsive to insulin and less effective at lowering your blood sugar back down to a normal level.

This forces your body to push out even more insulin until eventually you can no longer keep up and your blood sugar remains elevated. This is insulin resistance, a condition in which your body can no longer use insulin correctly and, according to Dr. Volk, the root cause of a lot of health issues.

The smart and easy way to optimize your metabolism is to say good-bye to sugar. You'll become a "fat burner" with ease as you reduce those carbohydrates.

When you reduce added sugars, you experience immediate and remarkable health benefits. And the fact is that almost all of us are affected by added sugars or are sensitive to a higher intake of carbohydrates. And if you're carb sensitive or carb intolerant (as 75 percent[2] of us are), it means that even foods like pastas and starchy carbohydrates can have a negative effect on your overall health.

How do you know if this applies to you? There are some identifiers that can help. Do you have trouble losing weight, or gain weight easily, or have higher markers that are indicative of metabolic syndrome (like waist circumference, higher blood sugar, high triglycerides, low HDL, and/or high blood pressure)? Even symptoms we do not always consider as part of or affecting our metabolism, such as trouble concentrating, constant bloating, or poor sleep, may all be related to some degree of carb sensitivity.

But if so many of us have issues with dietary carbohydrates, why is it repeatedly the main recommendation for seemingly "healthy" diets? Here the solution presents the challenge: half the battle is reducing carbs and the other half becomes adjusting the body to primarily rely on fats as fuel.

Once you find the right balance of high fat, moderate protein, and lower carbs—making sure not to go overboard on protein or skimp on fat because doing so results in more glucose—that's when your body can enter a state of nutritional ketosis.

**What happens when you're in nutritional ketosis:** A lot of good happens. Your body's metabolism comes into balance, you reduce inflammation, you feel better—and you reduce the risk of all those markers that make up metabolic syndrome, which, in turn, reduces the risk of disease.

Ketones have an incredible array of physiological benefits, including reduction of inflammation, reduction of body fat, and preserving lean muscle mass. I should also note that research suggests that ketones do more than just assist with energy. They may be involved with inflammation, immune function, brain metabolism, and may impact gut health.[3]

Scientifically, here's what's going on.

The moment you start a high-fat, low-carbohydrate diet, and as you stick with it, your body still seeks out sugar, so it taps into the glycogen stores in your muscles and liver (a stored form of glucose of about 2,000 calories). But once all that sugar is spent, it's left with no choice but to burn fat and create ketone bodies, an organic chemical compound made by your liver. This "fourth macronutrient" isn't present in the foods you eat. It's only when your body utilizes fat that you've eaten—or breaks down existing body fat—that it produces ketone bodies you can then use for energy. The more fat your body burns, the more ketones your body produces.

But the bigger picture—and what's interesting to experts like Dominic D'Agostino, Ph.D., researcher and associate professor at the University of South Florida who is considered the "king of keto," is how ketones have an effect on glucose. The more ketones you produce, the less blood sugar you have floating around, which means you're less likely to have metabolic trouble. Running on ketones has been shown to both suppress insulin and increase insulin sensitivity (how your body better manages insulin to reduce blood glucose). The more you can increase insulin sensitivity, the more you're able to decrease insulin resistance.

In conversations on this topic, Dr. D'Agostino indicates keeping insulin in check also helps you burn both stored body fat and the fat you eat for energy. It works like this: when you suppress insulin, it increases fat oxidation (the breaking down of fat for energy) and stimulates the expression of specific enzymes associated with fatty acid oxidation. So what you're doing, as Dr. D'Agostino puts it, is literally training your metabolism to use fat as an energy source and enhancing metabolic pathways associated with liberating fat from adipose tissue.

Some people *think* insulin sensitivity may improve when the body runs on ketones because most dieters run a calorie deficit in a state of nutritional ketosis. But Dr. D'Agostino was quick to point out that there is plenty of data to indicate that a ketogenic diet, and even ketone supplementation, can enhance insulin sensitivity by as much as 30 to 50 percent, independent of calorie restrictions.

If that is not good enough, we now know that ketones also act as signaling molecules and suppress inflammation in the body. The ketone metabolite beta-hydroxybutyrate (BHB) specifically blocks both the inflammatory pathway NF-kappaB and the NLRP3 inflammasome, two things that (when activated) trigger the release of pro-inflammatory cytokines. Beta-hydroxybutyrate is also one of the molecules that, by virtue of lowering inflammation, helps fundamentally change other metabolic pathways to promote greater fat oxidation, greater insulin sensitivity, and lower glucose—all of which are interrelated.

Science may have eventually come around to understand how omega-3s, monounsaturated fatty acids (MUFAs), and polyunsaturated fatty acids (PUFAs) are foundational to optimal health and need to be consumed regularly. But saturated fat? That's the one that still has a shadow over it, considered by many to be a leading contributor to major diseases. There are studies that appear to show that diets high in saturated fat correlate with a higher risk of cardiovascular disease.[4] But when researchers conducted a deeper analysis, they found that it's a diet high in both fat and carbohydrates that is most closely linked to cardiovascular disease. In fact, emerging evidence points to saturated fatty acids (SFAs) playing less of a role in coronary heart disease[5] than once thought, and that the consumption of added sugars may have a stronger association with the risk of coronary heart disease than SFAs.[6]

The latest data has been making experts question whether or not saturated fat has deserved such harsh scrutiny. They now see that if carbohydrate levels are low, higher saturated fat in the diet can lead to lower saturated fat in circulation, meaning that cholesterol and other metabolic markers will improve. For example, a 12-month trial found that subjects on a low-carb weight-loss diet who increased their percentage intake of dietary saturated fat improved their overall lipid profile and experienced a significant decrease in triglycerides and a modest increase in HDL cholesterol.[7] Some studies have tried increasing saturated fat several fold higher than the recommended amount and found that not only did subjects lose weight, but cholesterol panel and cardiometabolic health markers all uniformly improved.[8]

There's now evidence that when you switch from being a sugar burner to a fat burner, your metabolism of saturated fat may differ when you restrict carbohydrates. For example, research performed by Volk (and others) found that even doubling the amount of saturated fats in your diet doesn't elevate saturated fat in your blood when you're on a properly formulated low-carb diet.[9]

But that's not the only data overturning what we think we know about saturated fat. A recent study out of The Ohio State University fed subjects with metabolic syndrome three month-long controlled diets—a high-carb, a moderate-carb, and a low-carb diet (with a two-week break between diets).[10] Despite the fact that the low-carb diet contained two-and-a-half times more saturated fat than the high-carb diet, it decreased saturated fat in the bloodstream, and more than half of the participants watched their metabolic syndrome reverse.

**A state of keto-adaptation:** Ultimately, my goal is to help you get to the beginning stages of keto-adaptation—sustaining nutritional ketosis in a safe and optimal manner. You will usually be fat adapted metabolically within four to six weeks of consistent carb restriction. The research is very early in this area, but the potential is very exciting, in that it could have an effect on brain function, immune disorders, mental health, cancer, and more. In the long term it's keto-adaptation where we will see the big benefits.

But even in the beginning stages of the 22-day High Fiber Keto plan, similar to the women in the clinical study, you may experience many benefits, including:

- weight loss
- improvements in glucose, insulin sensitivity,[11] and blood pressure
- decrease in body fat
- improvements in sleep quality and energy
- reduced inflammation
- increased satiety and reduced cravings[12]

Many people struggle to see immediate results from a ketogenic diet. What many don't realize at the time is how we all produce ketones within a different time frame based on our unique biochemistry, our genetics, our lifestyle, and the stressors that enter and affect our lives. So you will likely have to experiment with your own preferences and body as you move past the first three weeks. The High Fiber Keto plan—the results of which are supported by a clinical study—is designed to help you succeed.

**How to measure nutritional ketosis:** While many think they are in nutritional ketosis because they have cut back carbs, the only way to truly feel confident is through blood tests. Now you can use home monitor kits to give you readings (the desired level is between 0.5 and 3.0 mmo/L).

**The challenges of entering nutritional ketosis:** Most people do find it difficult to get into nutritional ketosis. That can happen for a number of reasons—whether it's too much protein, too little fat, or even things like mineral imbalances. This is why the home monitor test is good, because you will be able to see if you are. It's also why I want you to stick to my 22-day plan, because it will provide the right nutritional ratios to help you get there.

And we also shouldn't neglect the fact that there can be other roadblocks that prevent you from getting there. They can be everything from lifestyle issues (is it the right time for you to undergo a major shift?) to other health considerations. Adopting a well-formulated ketogenic diet can be safe for many, but check with your medical provider beforehand as shifts in macronutrients, fluid balance, or electrolytes may interact with your health plan.

I will spend much of the rest of the chapter addressing common challenges and mistakes that people have when thinking about or trying to get into nutritional ketosis—with solutions for how you can approach them.

It's important to acknowledge that this will be a different approach for you, and it will likely have some challenges. That's one of the reasons why I ask you to be kind to your body (give yourself time to prepare, as I discuss in Chapter 8) and really think about developing some kind of social support to share in your struggles and join you in your joys.

The reality is that a ketogenic diet may offer the hope of weight loss, more energy and mental clarity, freedom from inflammation and cravings, and all of the benefits that can grant you an optimized metabolism.[13] Those benefits aren't always immediate. They are for most—but they definitely don't come to those who quit too soon. It has been more than two years for me, and the benefits are still coming. And that's why it's hugely important to prepare for both the challenges and common mistakes that come when you start keto.

## ATTACKING KETO'S BIGGEST CHALLENGES

As someone who didn't always get keto "right," I understand that making the switch can have its challenges. For me, the tough parts included overcoming a physical and psychological sugar addiction, getting enough electrolytes, staying hydrated, and eating "clean."

But those aren't the only difficulties. As you begin this journey, I want you to remember that it's okay if you don't get it perfectly right from the start (although I hope my 22-day plan will take the guesswork out of the transition). It may require some time for you to take the keto principles and put them into motion in the context of your daily life.

In addition, I don't want you to be surprised—and I don't want you to have preconceived notions about what some may chalk up to "keto roadblock." So I'll take you through some of the most common challenges that people face—and the ways that you can outsmart them.

## Some Say: It's too complex!

### Can-Do Keto: You only need to know one number.

While there are several versions of keto based on macronutrient breakdown, High Fiber Keto follows a relatively standard protocol of deriving 5 to 10 percent of your calories from carbohydrates, 20 to 25 percent from protein, and 65 to 75 percent from fat.

But here's the thing: you don't need to count anything or calculate any percentages. After learning the foods you eat, you'll naturally hit those general percentages, especially after doing my 22-day plan. The only number you'll ever need to keep an eye on is your ketone levels to make sure that you're always in a state of nutritional ketosis, which means your body is generating a level of ketones in a range of 0.5 to 3.0 mmol/L (15 to 300 mg/dL).[14] Although anywhere within this range is classically defined as being in nutritional ketosis, it seems 1.0 to 2.0mmol/L is the sweet spot for when those who are keto-adapted notice improvements beyond energy. For example, research and anecdotal evidence suggest people experience more mental sharpness, focus, concentration, energy, less inflammation, and some have reported improvement in skin. There are several ways to assess whether you have reached nutritional ketosis. To know that number, you have several options:

- You can use a breath analyzer. Being in nutritional ketosis causes an increase in the level of ketones in your breath. Breathing into one of these handheld devices gives you a measurement based on the acetones (a type of ketone) found in your breath.

- You can use over-the-counter urine strip kits that change color when saturated, indicating where your ketone levels are. (These kits are useful for the first few weeks of carbohydrate restriction but lose validity after two to four weeks).

- You can use a blood ketone meter, prick your finger, and place a small drop of blood on a contact strip to get a more accurate number. (The meter primarily assesses beta-hydroxybutyrate, or BHB).

Each method focuses on one of the three main ketone bodies. Each ketone plays a distinct role in the body, but the majority of research has focused on BHB, which seems to be linked to widespread and systemic effects on our bodies.

As of now, there's no sweet spot for an ideal number, according to Beth Zupec-Kania, R.D.N., C.D., a leading expert on nutritional ketosis. She suggests using your number more as a guide. And you'll have to take into consideration the time of day you take your measurement. For example, if you exercise (something as simple as taking a 30-minute walk) and then check your blood levels, your ketones naturally go down before they go up,[15] which can leave you feeling as if you're not accomplishing your goal.

## Some Say: The menu is too limited!

### Can-Do Keto: Pass the chocolate.

Yes, High Fiber Keto includes the tried-and-true healthy foods of fish, vegetables, olive oil, nuts, and seeds. But you will also enjoy meat, cheese, dairy, dark chocolate, berries, eggs, and even butter. In fact, many of the foods you're asked to stay away from are pretty much the same as those that most diets would have you avoid, such as processed fare, sugary foods (such as soda, candy, cakes, and fruit juices), and other items that otherwise have little to no nutritional value, like alcohol and various condiments.

## Some Say: Good luck sticking with it!

### Can-Do Keto: You just need to make it over the initial hump.

Yes, the first few weeks can be a difficult transition. In the first week, you can expect your body to react as it transitions out of relying on sugar for fuel, burns through its stored sugar (glycogen), and becomes accustomed to utilizing fat and ketones for energy. For some, that reaction can last for the first few days (and up to a few weeks) with symptoms that could include headaches, muscle cramps, constipation, diarrhea, general weakness, and rashes.[16] It's called the "keto flu," but with the following tips, these symptoms can be reduced or eliminated.

The good news is that with the help of leading keto researchers, my plan is specifically formulated to reduce—and in most cases even eliminate—keto flu by balancing your electrolytes, keeping you well hydrated, and maintaining the correct balance of the right types of fats.

Once you become fat adapted, many people actually find keto much easier to stick with than traditional diets. After a few weeks, you may find your carb cravings drastically reducing, or that you feel fuller and more satiated at each meal, and you'll notice you don't have the same hunger signals as when you run on carbohydrates. Instead of always feeling the urge to eat every two or three hours, you'll find yourself able to go between four and six hours. And because fat metabolizes more slowly than carbs, you'll also begin to enjoy all-day energy without experiencing any energy dips or hunger pangs, thanks to the steady levels of both blood sugar and insulin that a ketogenic diet allows.

Once you're fully keto-adapted (which for most takes around three to six weeks), as long as you continue to fuel your body with healthy fats, you'll be able to maintain a state of nutritional ketosis effortlessly and have a few more carbohydrates each day without them negatively influencing your ketone levels.

## Some Say: It's going to shock your system!

Can-Do Keto: Not if you prepare yourself properly.

Dr. Volk, who has worked with thousands of patients, has found that many people get so excited about the benefits of keto that they want to jump into the diet too quickly. This could mean not giving yourself any time to figure out the plan and prepare for what's to come (with your kitchen, your schedule, and prepping meals). That's why I developed my Pre-Fix Prep Plan to help you get ready. Don't underestimate the psychological and logistical switches that have to happen when you embark on a new nutrition plan. I'm as excited as you are for you to get started, but I don't want that excitement to come at the expense of being properly prepared for what's to come.

## Some Say: You can't break up with carbs!

## Can-Do Keto: You can step away from dysfunctional relationships.

As I mentioned earlier, I had a strong emotional and psychological addiction to sugar—thinking that I needed it at certain times to make me feel better. That's not uncommon since sweets and other carbs have long been popular comfort foods.

Indeed, the emotional impact that's made during the transition from burning sugar to fat is massive for many.[17] When Beth Zupec-Kania talks to patients, she compares carbs to alcohol for alcoholics. If you are addicted to carbohydrates—something Zupec-Kania believes most people are—the initial shock of giving them up can be distressing. Even if your body is able to make the transition without a hitch, your mind may keep you from staying the course because you're not looking at carbs as energy; you're eating them out of addiction.

She urges patients to realize how they need to change their relationship with food, starting with admitting that they are addicted to carbohydrates. Once you do that, it's key to then find a way to get past that without becoming miserable as a result, getting emotional, or feeling sorry for yourself. That's why my plan is set up to have you seek out support from others before you begin. By knowing how stepping away from carbs is going to affect you, and letting those around you know as well, you'll be able to break free from your carb addiction with less drama while your body switches over to fat and ketones.

**Some Say: You're going to eat the same foods over and over!**

**Can-Do Keto: No, you're not.**

It doesn't matter how delicious a diet might be, if it doesn't contain enough variety, you're going to bail because you're bored,[18] meaning you'll grab more food even though you're not hungry. You can counter this with more variety in your diet and by asking yourself if you're really still hungry. This is the reason I developed my plan to contain as many different meals as possible within a mere 22 days. It isn't simply because I want you to be excited by the menu; it's to make sure your body stays amazed as well.


## AVOIDING KETO'S BIGGEST MISTAKES

We all make mistakes. Every day. And while I don't believe that we should be in a constant state of chasing perfection, it is important to understand common mistakes that are made when following keto so you can optimize your metabolism and gain all of the health benefits from it. Here's how to avoid the common pitfalls when starting a keto lifestyle.

### Mistake: Forgetting the fat-protein friendship

When many follow a ketogenic diet, the spotlight is on fats and carbs—with protein serving as the understudy. That can be a big mistake, especially because so many keto beginners feel as if reaching often for more protein-rich foods (such as meats, nuts, and seeds) is a safe option because they're also rich in fats.

That mind-set can quickly get you into trouble, because any time you eat more protein than necessary to produce hormones, support healthy skin and hair, and build lean muscle, it triggers an insulin spike and turns all that extra protein into glucose (a process known as *gluconeogenesis*). This means that even if you're eating very few carbs, all that protein could be kicking your body out of nutritional ketosis. According to Volk, your level of daily protein should typically stay right at the standard recommended amount, which is exactly where my program is set.

## Mistake: Not drinking water wisely

Hydration isn't just fundamental for a healthy metabolism—it's critical for every single process that takes place within your body.[19] When your cells are adequately hydrated, each is able to function more optimally and efficiently, all of which influences what you're able to gain by being in nutritional ketosis. Despite this fact, so many people are walking around in a dehydrated state, according to Dr. Saenz. And when you're on a ketogenic diet, your need to stay hydrated only increases as your body begins to shed water that's attached to stored glycogen in your muscles.[20]

I start my day by adding a pinch of Himalayan salt to my water. I find it helps me with hydration. But for those on sodium-restricted diets, you should discuss your hydration needs with your doctor. As you reduce carbs, you release water (you may notice yourself going to the bathroom more in the first few days) and you may see some weight loss. But you're also losing sodium, so it's important to maintain hydration with water as well as with the salt.

Many of the symptoms of the "keto flu" (nausea, cramping, headaches, brain fog, sleep trouble) can actually be addressed by properly balancing sodium. (You may also need to add magnesium or potassium, which can be addressed with non-starchy fruits and vegetables.)

My program helps make it effortless for you to maintain the right balance of electrolytes required to stay adequately hydrated. It also incorporates plenty of water-rich foods that contain what is known as gel or *structured water*—the liquid found in plant and animal cells—which I've found can be a more efficient way to remain hydrated all day long.

## Mistake: Making it a free rein on fat— or fearing it all together

One of the biggest areas Dr. Volk sees some ketogenic dieters abuse is believing they can eat unlimited amounts of fat because they're now adapted. However, even just a little extra fat is still very calorically dense, so if you add more than your body needs to fuel itself—continually reaching for high-fat drinks or treats, thinking you're somehow immune—you can get into trouble fast.

Dr. Volk reminds patients that it's never an all-you-can-eat buffet in terms of fat just because you're now a fat burner. Just because you've switched fuel sources doesn't mean you're allowed to overfill your tank. You need to remind yourself that the fat you're using is a more efficient energy source, but when taken in amounts greater than what your body needs, it's still energy that can easily be stored.

On the flip side, it's important not to fear fat. Now, 65 to 75 percent of your diet will be fat; that's a big switch for most people who currently cover half their plate in carbs. But because fat is so dense (9 kilocalories per gram, compared to 4 kilocalories per gram for carbs), you can eat less food and have the same amount of satiety. My plan focuses on monounsaturated fats and saturated fats with smaller amounts of polyunsaturated fats to match recommended guidelines for essential fats in our diet.

## Mistake: Believing a cheat day is only a day

The term *cheat day* is something Dr. Volk dislikes because *cheat* means to gain an advantage. As she and other experts like to remind patients, adapting to nutritional ketosis can take weeks, and having that single cheat day can bring you right back to a place where it will take time to get back into nutritional ketosis.

Dr. Volk has encouraged patients to measure both their blood sugar and ketone levels before, during, and after a cheat day. Because when they do, the dramatic turn the numbers can take— blood sugar surging and ketones sinking—often speaks for itself.

But here's the thing: oftentimes that "need" to cheat is simply because you may crave something sweeter than you typically allow yourself to have, or you just feel you deserve something decadent in that moment. Satisfying that instant urge *without* throwing yourself out of nutritional ketosis is easily doable—if you have the right variety of sweet, rich desserts and snacks to turn to.

## Mistake: Assuming all fats are just fine

When I first began keto, I found myself eating a ton of nuts because they were high in "healthy" fats such as polyunsaturated fats (PUFAs) and so convenient. What I didn't know was that even when you're a fat burner, that doesn't necessarily mean any type of fat is optimal as fuel, according to Dr. Saenz.[21] One mistake many make is eating higher amounts of PUFAs, which are found in nearly all foods to a certain extent, but are richer in vegetable oils such as corn, soybean, sunflower, or cottonseed oil.

It makes sense in theory, since the two major classes of PUFAs—omega-3 fatty acids and omega-6 fatty acids—have been linked to improving symptoms in depression, anxiety, menstrual disorders, and yes, even metabolic syndrome.[22] These classes of fats are essential, says Volk, but with omega-6 fats, here's the catch: only in the amounts we need them.

She notes that when you switch over to a ketogenic diet, the amount of polyunsaturated fats that your body actually needs doesn't change. More is not necessarily better; in fact, eating too many omega-6 fats may cause cell damage and accelerate aging, since PUFAs (and other types of unsaturated fats) are technically unstable forms of fat that are prone to oxidation and have been shown to cause oxidative stress.[23] That's why the trick is not just eating more saturated and monounsaturated fats for fuel, but also keeping your polyunsaturated fat from rising.

## Mistake: Ignoring the micro

According to registered dietician Zupec-Kania, you could have your ratio of macros—your fats, proteins, and carbohydrates—in perfect order. However, it's the little details—certain individual nutrients responsible for tasks related to the protection or utilization of ketones—that can have the biggest effect on your body.

One example she shared involved a woman who had suffered from migraines and went on a ketogenic diet. She was the pinnacle of perfection when it came to maintaining a state of nutritional ketosis, yet her ketones mysteriously remained very low. Zupec-Kania checked for certain deficiencies and found her low in carnitine, a series of compounds that work at the cellular level to transport fatty acids.[24] Once supplemented with carnitine, the woman's ketone levels rose to exactly where they should have been in the first place. (My website NaomiWhittel.com has more details on micronutrients.)

Paying close attention to all of the micromanagers that work behind the scenes is just as important as keeping track of how much fat and protein and how many carbs you're taking in. For example, keto followers are more likely to have a mineral imbalance.[25] Inadequate amounts of sodium and magnesium are big ones, Volk says. People will recognize something is off and may even have a symptom (like an eye twitch, headaches, or a bedtime cramp), but they won't know that a magnesium deficiency likely is the root cause.

My program is therapeutically devised and nutrient comprehensive to make sure that you're not deficient in a particular compound or nutrient. For the most part, every single ingredient in every single recipe—right down to what may seem like a throwaway spice or herb—serves a purpose.

Of course, you may still have questions and might make some mistakes when trying out High Fiber Keto, but I've designed this 22-day plan to make it as error-proof as possible. But instead of your jumping in blindly, I'll guide you through the first three weeks to being fat adapted and on your way—not just using dietary fat but also maximizing my other favorite dietary f-word: *fiber*.

### Ready? Get Set, Go!

My 22-day plan and the time you spend preparing beforehand will give you all the info you need to get going on your High Fiber Keto journey. But if you're at the point where you're getting ready to make a change, there are a few things you can do right now to mentally prepare.

1. Make sure you have a support system—whether it's a friend or family member. You will be much better equipped to transition when you have someone or a group of people you can lean on for support.

2. Organize your household. This does require a bit of time. Address your pantry and fridge and remove the foods that aren't keto-friendly. Creating the right environment is one of the keys to success.

3. Remember that each person has a different carb-fat ratio and experience of nutritional ketosis. You may have to experiment a bit and really get in tune with when you're feeling satiated and good, using the objective numbers to figure out when you feel best and trend toward a healthier profile.

4. Take some time for yourself. Your own personal mind-set will be the number one determinant of your success. Spend some time thinking about what you want, your current lifestyle, and what you can do. When your mind is ready, your body will follow.

# LINDSAY

### I got control of my life—and my eating.

One year after I had my fourth child, I was having trouble getting the weight off. And I didn't even realize how many carbs I was having every day. I knew I was eating them because they're fast and easy. I just didn't feel good.

So I went into High Fiber Keto with one goal—just to see if I could stick with it and see what it did for me. And what I found was amazing. Yes, I was craving some carbs and sugar (even when I wasn't hungry), and I had some trouble getting enough fat early on (going low carb wasn't hard at all). But it only took a week for those cravings to go away. No more highs and lows, and I felt better than I ever had before.

I had energy. I didn't feel foggy. And my blood sugar levels were spectacular—in the 90s in the morning and, by the end of the program, steadily in the low 80s and 70s. I lost 3 percent body fat in 21 days! I have continued this lifestyle. I'm down 10 pounds, 145 to 135. The weight is still coming off, and I went from size 8 to size 4.

But the best part was that I got control of my life—and my eating.

# CHAPTER THREE

# FIBER: THE KEY TO KETO

## The Secret to Maximizing Keto and Optimizing Your Metabolism

This is the great oxymoron, right? Fiber and keto?

After all, it seems like a natural question: If keto is a carb-restrictive diet, then why would keto include fiber? How does it fit in?

At first glance, they might seem like archenemies rather than a dynamic duo. How could a plan centered around fat include such a carb-centric nutrient like fiber? I get it. When I first started exploring keto, the low-carb sirens went off. Fiber—so often associated with such foods as beans, oatmeal, and whole-grain breads—doesn't *feel* keto. In fact, it feels like the exact opposite. *One serving of black beans? Not a chance! It will take me out of nutritional ketosis!*

But what we have learned serves as the key to making High Fiber Keto work for you. So much of succeeding in health and life is about making quick switches—small adjustments that make big differences. This is what High Fiber Keto is all about, establishing your foundational keto diet to turn your body into a fat-burning system and then integrating the nuance of fiber into your overall nutritional approach to optimize your metabolism.

The big myth about keto is that keto should restrict fiber. It's the exact opposite. A keto diet should be designed with non-starchy veggies, nuts, seeds, and fruits, totaling about 30 to 50 grams a day, with about 20 grams of fiber every day. This chapter is all about taking you through the importance of fiber, how it works, and how it needs to be a part of your keto diet to maximize your health.

I have been keto for about two years—sometimes making mistakes, sometimes hitting a groove—but not until I made this quick switch of adding more fiber to my keto diet did I really find my better health, better metabolic markers, and a much better sense of wellness and energy.

The evidence in fiber's favor is overwhelming. We're simply not getting enough, even though fiber is such an important determinant of good health outcomes.

Fiber is a nutritional firefighter. Sure, you know it's there, but you probably take it for granted until the moment you need it. And that's when you realize what power and influence it really has. And considering the metabolic health crisis that we're currently in, I'd say the five-alarm fire raging in our bodies needs our attention. It certainly did in mine. Fiber—if you call on it to help—can protect and heal you.

Too often, because keto lifestyle followers tend to be so focused on dietary fat, we inadvertently ignore other important nutrients. Part of what I have done with my 22-day plan is to integrate fiber in the right amounts and in the right ways, so you can enjoy the benefits while still staying in nutritional ketosis. That is, it's not about eating whole grains, which can be inflammatory for most people, but rather consuming your fiber in keto-friendly ways.

In my plan, I've carefully selected the highest fiber options, such as artichokes, non-starchy vegetables, cruciferous vegetables, avocados, nuts, coconuts, and seeds such as chia seeds and flaxseeds. In this chapter, I'll take you through the power and potential of fiber by outlining my five favorite fiber facts. You'll see how to combine fiber and keto for the most health-boosting benefits.

# FIBER FACT ONE

## A Fiber Deficiency Prevents You from Being Optimally Healthy

For so long, fiber has been the nutritional runt of the litter: it gets ignored a lot.

Consider this alarming stat: roughly 9 out of 10 of us do not get enough fiber in our diets, which means that there's a 90 percent chance that you are fiber deficient.[1] And even though women over 50 in this country seem to be much smarter about eating more fiber, only 15 percent actually take in the recommended amount.

Fiber has been identified as a "nutrient of concern" since 2005 because so many of us are deficient, which places us at a serious metabolic disadvantage and must be addressed. If we increased fiber by just 3 grams per day, it would save $2 billion in medical costs associated with constipation alone![2]

The fiber gap likely happened because of the heavy reliance on sugary food in today's common diet. When food is processed, fiber is typically the first nutrient to be removed. Many leaders in conventional medicine will argue that when you remove gluten or grains from the diet (which is becoming a more common approach for treating inflammatory conditions), you will be losing important fiber. This can certainly be the case *if* those whole grains are being replaced by processed food. It's worth noting here that many also make the assumption that the best and only way to get fiber is through whole grains. That's not the case, as my plan will outline.

Why is this fiber deficiency such a problem? Because fiber truly is a super-nutrient. This health hero works throughout your body to fight more conditions than you probably realize.

Let's consider the data. A wealth of evidence from more than 240 studies and trials across 40 years of research suggests fiber will reduce your risk of coronary heart disease, type 2 diabetes, colorectal cancer, and even premature death between 7 and 19 percent.[3,4] It's so powerful that it can help with satiety and weight management. It can reduce the risk of metabolic syndrome and other cardiometabolic risks, including cardiovascular inflammation and obesity[5] and it can also nourish your microbiome (the microorganisms living in the body that influence so much of our health) and your immune system and support overall metabolism.

Simply put, by getting the right amount of dietary fiber into your diet, the less risk you will have of experiencing metabolic syndrome because of fiber's ability to lower blood sugar, blood pressure, triglycerides, and belly fat—as well as LDL (the "bad" cholesterol).[6]

One of the most comprehensive meta-analyses (a statistical analysis of multiple scientific studies) ever performed on the nutrient looked at 185 observational studies and 58 clinical trials that were conducted during a 40-year period. These studies looked at various factors in diet, including fiber and quality of carbohydrates. This research funded by the World Health Organization showed that high consumption of dietary fiber is associated with a 15 to 31 percent reduced risk of coronary heart disease, stroke, type 2 diabetes, colorectal cancer, and all-cause and cardiovascular-related death.[7] In fact, every 8-gram increase of daily fiber was associated with a 7 to 19 percent reduced risk of coronary heart disease, type 2 diabetes, colorectal cancer, and death.

For women, the recommended daily intake of fiber is between 21 and 25 grams, or 21 grams if over the age of 50.[8] But when I spoke with Dr. Mike Hoaglin, M.D., physician executive and clinical microbiome expert, he shared the fact that most people don't come close to that amount. On average, most people worldwide eat fewer than 20 grams a day,[9] and in the United States, that number drops even lower to about 17 grams per day.[10]

In my plan, you're going to get to the optimum amounts—while encouraging fat adaptation and nutritional ketosis—so you can enjoy the double-dose benefits of a High Fiber Keto life.

# FIBER FACT TWO

## Fiber Influences Many Bodily Systems

Fiber is essentially a carbohydrate that your body can't digest because it doesn't have the enzymes, and it comes in two forms. (See how fiber moves through your digestive system on page 54.) Both types of fiber are important for healthy and regular digestion, and most veggies, fruits, nuts, and seeds contain fiber.

| Fiber | Action | Forms |
| --- | --- | --- |
| Insoluble | Does not dissolve in water, helps push stool through the colon | • Beta glucans found in mushrooms and seaweed<br>• Cellulose and hemi-cellulose found in all plant cell walls; lettuce, broccoli, cauliflower, and the rest of the non-starchy vegetables are good sources<br>• Lignins found in seeds |
| Soluble | Soluble in water; makes you feel fuller longer by providing bulk in the digestive system; fermentable by bacteria in the colon | • Inulin found in foods like chicory root and artichokes<br>• Pectin found in berries and tomatoes<br>• Alginic acids found in algae |

As you increase the fat in your diet and decrease carbohydrates, there's less room for some of the high-fiber foods that you used to rely on as your go-to fiber sources. But that's all the more reason why you need to pay special attention to fiber as you begin your keto diet. It's easy to ignore it, but you shouldn't. Why? Besides the disease outcomes just discussed, fiber plays a special role because of the way it interacts with and influences many systems in the body.

**Fiber balances blood sugar.** You already know High Fiber Keto is going to help you balance blood sugar because your body will primarily be using fat for fuel. Fiber itself also helps regulate blood sugar. You'll still be getting small amounts of carbohydrates in your meals (fewer than 50 grams of total carbohydrates per day), but the fact that a high percentage of your carbohydrates are fiber-rich is why your blood sugar after meals will be even more balanced.

**Fiber helps with satiety.** When you transition from a higher carbohydrate diet to a keto diet, you may feel that your plate doesn't look as full. Why? Higher fat foods are denser and don't take up as much room on your plate. But because fat is very filling, you will feel full with less food. When you add in the higher-fiber foods, you will also add volume, which will help to create the visual cue that you are eating a full plate of food. If you are used to filling your plate with grains, bread products, legumes, and fruits, replacing those foods with keto-approved, fiber-rich foods will be your best substitution. The added bonus, of course, is that these will also take up volume in your stomach and help contribute to your feeling of satiety that you're already feeling with a high-fat diet.

**Fiber decreases cravings.** Lower cravings go hand-in-hand with increased satiety. When you are more satisfied from your meal, you are less likely to go for something sweet directly after eating or feel hungry again in an hour. Since fiber helps to balance blood glucose, you get the bonus of decreased cravings. Your blood sugar won't spike after a meal only to drop again an hour later and cause you to go searching for the next sugary thing to eat.

Blood sugar is also balanced via your microbiome. By feeding the beneficial bacteria, soluble and prebiotic fiber can essentially change the composition of the bacteria. One theory in nutrition science is that it isn't you that craves sugar; it is *your microbiome*. This certainly makes sense since when the microbiome is out of balance, there may be more organisms that run on sugar and other processed carbohydrates. By eating more fiber, you may effectively crowd out these less desirable bacteria.

**Fiber-rich foods are nutrient-dense foods.** The plant foods in your High Fiber Keto plan are all in their whole, unrefined state. Along with the blast of fiber, you will be getting vitamins, minerals, essential fats, and a host of phytonutrients, such as carotenoids, resveratrol, and flavonoids that support metabolism, reduce inflammation, and keep your body functioning at its optimal level.

Nutrient density is absolutely fundamental in gaining your optimized metabolism. It takes a lot of nutrients for each body system to function, and if you are low in even just one micronutrient, let alone several, it limits what your body is capable of. Food is always the first place I recommend finding fiber and nutrients, and then supplementation can help to fill in any gaps and optimize your metabolism and health.

**Fiber helps with digestion issues.** Anytime the body undergoes a big change in diet, particularly when shifting from a low-fat or Standard American Diet to a ketogenic diet, it may take a few days for your digestion to adjust. When your body isn't breaking down food efficiently, constipation (or sometimes loose, oily stools) may be the result. This most often happens because of a sodium imbalance. Adding high-fiber, keto-approved foods will assist with regulating your digestion.

Not only is constipation uncomfortable, from a metabolic perspective, it can impact how effectively your body absorbs nutrients from food. Regular elimination through the colon is important, as it is one route that the body can get rid of waste. As your metabolism shifts from sugar burning to fat burning, your body will undergo detoxification, and these toxins will need to get out of the body. Constipation can also contribute to "keto flu."

Insoluble fiber—along with making sure your sodium stays high—helps to keep things moving through the digestive system and creates bulk in the stool. Soluble fiber, and especially prebiotics, provides a food source to the beneficial bacteria in the colon, which helps to regulate bowel movements.

## *Fiber: How It's Digested*

**In the mouth:** Chewing and enzymes in the saliva work to break fiber away from the other components in the food, including digestible carbohydrates, vitamins, minerals, and plant compounds such as polyphenols. Salivary amylase is the main enzyme in saliva that works to break down the digestible carbohydrates. Also, smelling, seeing, tasting, and chewing are very important parts of the digestive process because they help to prime your digestive tract to receive food, meaning that digestion begins even before food enters the mouth.

**In the stomach:** Hydrochloric acid and pepsin (a digestive enzyme) work to digest proteins, further releasing the fiber from the rest of the components in the food. The stomach muscles churn and food is further broken down, resulting in chyme, a liquid substance made of stomach juices and partially digested food.

**In the small intestine:** Pancreatic enzymes and intestinal enzymes break protein, carbohydrates, and fat into their smallest components. Starches break down into glucose, proteins into amino acids, and fats into fatty acids. These nutrients, along with micronutrients (vitamins and minerals), are then absorbed into the body. Bile is released by the gallbladder to help you digest and absorb fat. The fiber becomes separate from the other food components. Soluble fiber will absorb some water.

**In the large intestine/colon:** Prebiotic fiber is fermented by probiotic bacteria to create short-chain fatty acids (such as butyric acid), vitamin $B_{12}$, vitamin $K_2$, and other important compounds that can then be absorbed into the body or used by the cells in the colon. Fiber that isn't probiotic remains largely unchanged and will make up the bulk of the stool when it is excreted.

## FIBER FACT THREE

### The Secret Fiber Weapon Is Called Butyrate

One of the biggest arguments against keto is how lacking it can be in fiber, which, by design, makes perfect sense. Switching from being a sugar burner to a fat burner—and getting your liver to adjust from utilizing carbohydrates and synthesizing fatty acids to producing ketone bodies and oxidizing fatty acids—requires eating a variety of high-fat, low-carb foods such as avocado, nuts, seeds, butter, coconut oil, or MCT oil.

It's that strict ratio of fats versus carbs that oftentimes pushes out the possibility of getting enough fiber in your day, since many traditional high-fiber foods such as grains (rice, quinoa, and oats, for example), beans and legumes, various fruits (including apples, dates, and pears), and certain veggies (like sweet potatoes) all contain abundant amounts of starches and sugar that quickly kick you out of nutritional ketosis.

Each time I asked "the fiber question," I was met with a variety of conflicting answers:

- "It's impossible to eat plenty of fiber and stay in ketosis!"
- "You don't need to eat as much fiber when on keto!"
- "Just add a fiber supplement to your diet, and you'll be fine!"
- "I'm smart about eating enough fiber when on keto—so I'm fine!"

So why are so many conflicted about this subject? If fiber is just as vital for creating an optimized metabolism as a ketogenic diet, why would anyone ever consider removing such an asset from their metabolic arsenal? More importantly, is it *actually* possible to find harmony between these two game changers to allow you to achieve a more efficient metabolism?

The answer, of course, is yes. And it primarily revolves around a compound you may have never heard about.

It's called *butyrate*, and it's a superhero within its fatty acid community.

Butyrate is a short-chain fatty acid (SCFA). Produced in the colon and from fiber, SCFAs have three main actions centered around gut health, energy, and your immune system. Butyrate is a common SCFA made from fiber, and it is involved in energy production, the immune system, and regulating inflammation. Butyrate is essential for digestive health.

High-fiber foods such as leafy greens and asparagus enable butyrate-producing bacteria to thrive. We can also obtain butyrate in the form of butyric acid through our diet, mainly from creamy, rich, grass-fed butter (the term *butyrate* actually derives from the Greek word for butter). According to studies, one tablespoon of butter typically delivers 14 grams of fat, of which 560 mg is butyric acid.[11]

Butyrate has many health benefits, including increased insulin sensitivity, improved cardiovascular health, lower cholesterol, reduced inflammation,[12] and better appetite control. Butyrate may also be capable of increasing mitochondrial activity,[13] a new area of research that, if found in humans, may indicate increased energy and reduce ROS. That's because butyrate is similar in structure to a ketone body that can be used by the mitochondria for fuel; it's called *beta-hydroxybutyrate*.

The butyrate-producing function of fiber further enhances its importance as part of the ketogenic diet. While it used to be easy to ignore fiber's value, there is now too much evidence of its importance to discount it anymore.

# FIBER FACT FOUR

## Fiber Helps Feed Your All-Important Microbiome

You've already learned a lot about your microbiome and how it's affected by fiber and keto. This is such a huge topic, however, that it qualifies for an in-depth explanation. There's a complex community of trillions of microorganisms (bacteria, fungi, and viruses) living inside you that collectively make up your *microbiome*. They exist everywhere, including your skin, mouth, nose, vagina, and most importantly for metabolic health, your intestines (or gut microbiome). But you don't start out with all those microorganisms all at once.

You get your first mix of microbes from your mother. Thanks, Mom! Then how you are born, either vaginally or by cesarean section, determines which kinds of microbes move in next. After that, you're pretty much a walking magnet for microbes for the rest of your life. Everything that happens to you and everything you're exposed to—from disease, stress, injuries, illness, and antibiotics to puberty, pregnancy, and menopause—can change what colonizes your body.[14] But there's something else that plays a big part in what lives inside you, and that's the food you eat.

When you're an infant, you have about 100 different species of bacteria inside your gut.[15] But by the time you're an adult, there are more than 1,000 types of bacteria living there—some good and some bad. The good bacteria do everything from assisting with food digestion and increasing the production of antibodies to training your immune system to attack pathogens throughout your entire body. These intestinal microbes even make vitamins that you can't make on your own, such as $B_{12}$,[16] which helps with red blood cell formation, lowers your risk of anemia, and keeps both your nerves and blood cells healthy.

What's so interesting to me is that any change in the foods we eat directly affects our gut microbes and changes the ratio of both good and bad bacteria.[17] Eat the right mixture of foods, and the good bacteria stay in charge. But when things are out of balance in our bodies—which can happen when we don't eat a diverse enough diet—even the subtlest changes to that microbial community can lead to conditions and diseases from the nonlethal (such as acne, eczema, and cavities) to the life threatening (such as obesity, hardening of the arteries, diabetes, autoimmune disease, and cancer).[18] In fact, experts believe that our gut health affects 90 percent of our immune system's functions![19]

With all that responsibility placed on those tiny tenants inside us, you can see why keeping them well fed with the right amounts of fiber and the perfect blend of microbiome-supportive nutrients is absolutely critical to metabolic health. But don't despair. If you are getting down on yourself for not eating enough fiber or not having the "perfect" diet, remember this: on your High Fiber Keto plan, your microbiome will shift in a matter of *days*. Good nutrition works *that* fast!

And fiber is going to be one of your smartest tools to improve both the quantity of beneficial bacteria and the balance of different organisms.

While new and exciting research is becoming available, the scientific field already recognizes that:

**More diversity is always better:** It's understood that a more diverse microbiome is better,[20] meaning that the more types, species, and strains of microorganisms you host, the more balanced and healthier your microbiome will be.

**You—or rather, *they*—are what you eat:** Your gut microbiome is directly affected by food, and research has revealed that within as little as a few days—or perhaps even sooner, after almost every meal—changes that reflect what you just ate can be seen in the microbiome.[21] And it's these little changes that can directly affect your health—for better or for worse.

### A Prebiotics Primer

We can't really talk about fiber without talking about prebiotics—compounds that become favorite foods for probiotics, the beneficial bacteria that make up our microbiome. Prebiotics can improve the composition, amount, and activity of the probiotics. When we consume prebiotics, the probiotics can do more of what they do to support our health, including creating beneficial compounds and crowding out pathogens. Most prebiotics are types of fiber, but prebiotics can also include polyphenols, my favorite antioxidant found in foods such as berries, red wine, and green tea, and there are likely many other compounds with prebiotic effects that scientists have yet to identify. Here are the keto prebiotics:

| Prebiotic | Classification | Description | Keto Food Sources |
|---|---|---|---|
| Inulin | Soluble fiber, fructan; can be synthetically derived from chicory root | Most common type of prebiotic found in plants, along with FOS. Inulin improves digestion, balances the microbiome, supports healthy metabolic function, prevents chronic disease.[22] | Asparagus, burdock, burdock root, chicory root, dandelion greens, garlic, Jerusalem artichokes, jicama, leeks, onions |
| Fructo-oligosaccha-rides (FOS) | Soluble fiber; can be synthetically produced and used in food products because of its sweet flavor | Often found in the same plants as inulin. Improves digestion, balances the microbiome, supports healthy metabolic function, prevents chronic disease. | Artichoke, aspar-agus, burdock root, chicory root, garlic, Jerusalem artichokes, jicama, leeks, onions, |
| Galacto-oligosaccha-rides (GOS)[23] | Soluble fiber; most is synthetically pro-duced and contains some lactose and glucose; a GOS-like compound is found in human breast milk[24] | GOS is often used in sup-plements/treatments for constipation and is added to infant formulas. | |
| Resistant Starch | Insoluble fiber, but functions more like soluble fiber; types 1, 2, and 3 from dietary fiber; type 4 is syn-thetically produced | Resistant starch has been shown to improve metabolic health and the microbiome. See below for a detailed discussion. | Green bananas, green plantains, potato starch, seeds, cooked and cooled white rice or potatoes |
| Lactulose | Synthetically pro-duced from lactose (milk sugar) | Prescription solution used in the lactulose breath test to diagnose small intestine bacterial overgrowth (SIBO) where the colon micro-biome has migrated into the small intestine. Used clinically as a treatment for constipation and high ammonia in the blood. | |
| Polyphenols[25] | Not fiber, but have prebiotic activity | Polyphenols are com-pounds that give plants their color and often act as antioxidants. | Black tea, blueber-ries and other types of berries, cacao,[26] coffee, flaxseeds, green tea, onions, spinach |

# FIBER FACT FIVE

## Fiber Is Keto-Friendly!

Your High Fiber Keto meal plan *is* high in fiber, even though most people out there thought it was impossible to do! My team of Ph.D.s and nutritionists helped me ensure that we use good fats and enough protein to meet your needs while keeping total carbohydrates under 50 grams per day.

What I've found in my life, and translated for you in the meal plan, is that high-fiber plant foods are essential to your diet. Many of these foods, including Jerusalem artichokes, dandelion greens, artichokes, and asparagus, also contain prebiotic fibers. Depending on its size, a single medium artichoke has more fiber than any other vegetable, which is why it has become one of my favorite foods.

By following your High Fiber Keto plan, you may actually be eating *more* fiber than you were before keto and will definitely consume more than the average person. Once you get the hang of building your plate using the bulk and volume of these non-starchy, fiber-rich foods, meeting your fiber needs will hardly take any thought at all.

The main reason I've seen fiber become so feared by many keto dieters is that certain high-fiber foods that are also high-carb foods are assumed to be automatically discounted from the keto plan.

Surgeon and diet-microbiome researcher Victoria Gershuni, M.D., MTR, MSGM, described how many of her patients walk away from the most obvious of healthy foods—green leafy vegetables— because they worry about being kicked out of nutritional ketosis. She explained that initially you do have to be more rigid about eating carbohydrates from vegetables as your body begins to switch over to an alternative fuel source because you don't have as much mitochondrial enzyme capacity as you need to produce ketones.

However, as you stay in nutritional ketosis, you simultaneously teach your mitochondria to utilize fat for fuel, which in turn increases your mitochondrial enzyme capacity. As that rises, you can gradually increase your carb intake without being bumped out of nutritional ketosis. Note that fluctuations throughout the day and from day to day are normal, and you don't necessarily always need to have really high ketone levels, as more isn't always better.

Ultimately, your body will become a keto-adapted, fat-burning machine. This 22-day journey is about setting you up to shift to fat adaptation, knowing that you don't have to give up fiber to do so. In fact, they are a dynamic duo.

## SUSANNAH

### I felt leaner through my lower abdominals and hips.

I've tried other diets, like Whole30, and I've always been interested in and considered keto. But I never gave it a try until this study.

The best part about it? I had more consistent, even energy throughout the day and didn't feel jumpy in the morning or tired in the afternoon. I was better able to cope with daily stress. I found that my mental clarity seemed better—I could organize and multitask much more efficiently at work and at home.

Plus, there were some other benefits, like better-looking skin and a better-feeling body. I didn't have significant weight-loss goals, but I felt leaner after a month on the program, especially through the lower abdominals and hips.

I did have some food cravings early on for the sugar and carbs I'm used to, but they faded quickly, and I never felt hungry or unsatisfied on this plan. The truth is, I actually felt *more* satisfied after eating. I attribute this to the good fats I consumed through-out the program. And the salty foods—pickles and olives—felt like a luxury. Plus, I loved how the butter and oil are so satisfying.

CHAPTER **FOUR**

# YOUR *WISH* LIST

## The Long and the Short of It

For better or worse, many of us operate in instant-gratification mode. We can't stand being stuck in traffic. We get frustrated when the Wi-Fi is slow. And don't even talk to us if four people are ahead of us in the coffee line. Maybe it's simply an offshoot of our technological advances and our gotta-keep-moving culture, but patience can be difficult to manage for sure.

That's also true when it comes to health and the transformation you likely want to see once you start making behavioral changes. When it comes to putting your body at an optimized metabolism, those changes can start quickly, but you may not see all of them right away (namely, because many shifts require a blood test to confirm).

Ultimately, the goal of High Fiber Keto is to help give you the greatest possible optimized metabolism—to take control of the factors that make up metabolic syndrome. But while you are working toward your long-term goal of optimizing your metabolism, I'm also very aware that you have shorter-term concerns as well.

In fact, there's likely one thing that ultimately drives everything you do in your day-to-day life, and that is how you *feel*.

And you know what? It's okay to not feel much patience. Maybe you've tried lots of different programs and approaches, maybe you're frustrated that you can't sync your body to do what your mind wants to do, or maybe you're just frustrated that you're living in first or second gear when you really want to be in fourth or fifth.

Consider that (1) an estimated 75 percent of the world's population is carb-intolerant,[1] (2) 90 percent of Americans are deficient in fiber,[2] and (3) your 38 trillion bacteria may not have the most beneficial makeup (note: the number of bacteria is slightly higher than the number of cells that make up your body, which at last count, totaled 30 trillion[3]).

Those factors can manifest themselves in a number of ways— low energy, mood swings, fatigue, weight gain, hormonal imbalances, and so many other factors.

It's no wonder that you wish for something big to happen— and as quickly as possible.

That's one of the main reasons why I designed this plan: to help you overcome struggles that so many people face every day. In particular, there are four areas of our life where we yearn for control, with the hope of not just *being* healthier, but *feeling* healthier, too:

- **W**eight imbalance
- **I**mperfect skin
- **S**tress and anxiety
- **H**ormones

The good news is that when you switch over from being a sugar burner to a fat burner and become keto-adapted, WISH starts to become your reality.

The best means for WISH to come healthily true is a well-balanced diet. This allows you to bring the widest possible variety of high-fat, fiber-rich, low-carb foods to your table in a way that will satisfy you and transport the greatest variety of bacteria and other microorganisms to your gut microbiome.

That's why High Fiber Keto has these components:

- The right balance of high-fat, low-carb foods that make it easiest to get into—and stay in—nutritional ketosis

- The right fats to support nutritional ketosis and all the cells of your body

- The right ratio of soluble and insoluble fiber in their purest forms to maximize your metabolic benefits and allow you to boost butyrate production even further than keto does alone

- The right mixture of nutrients that both sustain your microbiome and feed the good bacteria within it so they can flourish

Now, before I go over the four things on this WISH list—weight loss, improved skin, stress reduction, and hormonal balance—it's important to understand where all of these issues originate: in your brain.

Sara Burke, Ph.D., associate professor in the department of neuroscience at the University of Florida, says that making improvements in these WISH list categories begins with your brain. When we talk about brain health, most people just assume this means being able to think more clearly, as well as retaining and remembering things better. But that's just a small portion of the total body benefits that immediately come from improving your brain health. All the things on our WISH list—weight control, improved skin, stress reduction, and hormonal balance—all tie back to your brain.

The brain weighs, on average, a mere three pounds, yet it takes up 20 percent of our metabolic resources.[4] It's the most important organ in our body, the control center that manages every single bodily process. And if it's not operating as efficiently as possible, then nothing is operating as efficiently as possible.

The brain is the CEO of your body, and every single cell within it is an employee. Your brain runs the show by telling your cells what to do and when to do it, making sure that they are doing their job. Business booms when everyone listens and everything gets done.

But when your brain decides to hang out on Twitter instead of multi-tasking, or it can't make the right decisions fast enough, production suffers, scared stockholders start jumping ship, and business grinds to a disastrous halt.

So in order to best maximize your overall health, you have to make sure that your CEO is working well. When you follow a lifestyle that maximizes brain function, such as proper cardiovascular fitness, getting enough sleep, and eating a high-fiber ketogenic diet, everything falls into place, according to Dr. Burke.

Your brain primarily runs on glucose and when you follow a carb-dominant diet, it runs almost exclusively on glucose. That makes your mind more subject to the energy peaks and valleys that relying on carbs can cause. Add the fact that as your ability to transport glucose declines with age (due to producing less estrogen), your brain becomes even more susceptible to not running at an even, highly efficient pace.

But your brain is also able to utilize ketones, the only other fuel the brain will use for energy. When you follow a diet that encourages nutritional ketosis, your brain can use a mixture of glucose and ketones for energy, making for a steadier flow of energy no longer at the mercy of the smaller stores of glucose and available via the higher levels of fat breakdown. Because the brain can rely on another fuel source, it can preserve glucose for other functions. This prevents your brain from experiencing any energy ebbs and flows, since your body is capable of holding up to (and using to create ketones when necessary) roughly 40,000-plus calories worth of fat. It's this instant access to energy that Dr. D'Agostino believes helps prevent metabolism imbalances that can occur with sugar burners when their brain cells are either starved of (or have difficulty processing) glucose.

Note: As a further testament to its impact on the brain, a ketogenic diet has also been shown to be effective at managing epilepsy, as well as showing great promise with other neurological issues, including sleep disorders, anxiety, Parkinson's, and even Alzheimer's. Part of its efficacy goes back to its ability to reduce chronic inflammation.

In other words, as your brain becomes healthier, your body follows suit. And that's when you start to feel differences in your health—not just because of what your blood tests show, but how you feel in your everyday life.

In this chapter, we'll look closely at the four main areas of your WISH list, beginning with the first item on the list.

## WEIGHT LOSS AND MAINTENANCE (AND BETTER BODY COMP)

The number one reason many people seek out a keto-based lifestyle is weight loss. And when you establish a metabolic ketone marriage fueled with good fat, fiber, and a balanced microbiome, this goal not only becomes easier to obtain, the results can go beyond what you expect or ever thought you'd achieve.

One important note: weight loss, while very common on keto, doesn't happen for everyone. Yes, placing your body in the state of nutritional ketosis helps lower blood sugar, burns off excess fat, and lets your body utilize more of the fats you're consuming for fuel—all of which can lead to weight loss for life. But as I mentioned before, if you're not specifically eating a well-formulated ketogenic diet, you can easily consume more calories than your body requires. You also can miss out on specific essential nutrients, placing yourself at a nutritional disadvantage that can slow down your metabolism and impair other key processes related to food metabolization.

Other factors that cause many on keto to come to a crashing weight-loss halt include dealing with chronic stress (which can cause the body to store fat[5]), lack of physical activity, and not getting enough sleep.[6] These may sound like obvious roadblocks, but according to researchers and the comments I've received from many of you, most people make two major mistakes when it comes to keto and weight loss:

First, they expect a ketogenic diet to take care of everything for them—meaning, they don't think about other aspects of their life that may benefit from changing. And second, they try to do too much exercise, which can cause the body to burn out a lot sooner, especially early on as it adjusts to switching to fat as a fuel source.

High Fiber Keto takes these tendencies into account to help you maximize the chances of improving your body composition with a high-fiber ketogenic diet.

- Each day's menus are therapeutically designed and nutrient-comprehensive, so you're never left hungry or at a nutritional disadvantage.

- It is effective at reducing stress, helping your body to be far less likely to hold on to any fat you're trying to shed.

- You'll be getting plenty of physical activity by following a metabolic movement plan that's excuse-proof and tailored to your fitness level, allowing you to improve your metabolism and burn more fat without burning out.

- It corrects an imbalance in electrolytes (commonly caused by poorly formulated ketogenic diets) that has been shown to disrupt sleep.

## IMPERFECT SKIN

No matter our skin goal—whether it is radiating a youthful, fresh appearance or erasing fine lines—we could all use a program that could prevent several of the skin-related issues that plague us.

Reducing your sugar intake through a ketogenic diet has a tremendous positive effect on your skin. Studies continue to demonstrate that a diet high in sugar can contribute to acne,[7] and those who suffer from moderate to severe acne typically consume greater amounts of carbohydrates.[8] However, keeping your insulin levels low using High Fiber Keto diminishes the excess production of oil and helps your pores go from clogged to clear! It does this by minimizing the release of insulin-like growth factor 1 (IGF-1), a hormone shown to cause complexion problems through raising sebum production.[9]

Dr. Volk shared with me how she had personally witnessed allergies, rashes, and other skin irritations clear up in patients who were on a ketogenic diet.

One of the biggest issues that High Fiber Keto alleviates is insulin aging you by being cruel to your collagen, the beauty protein that acts as the support structure for your skin. Every time your body has an insulin surge due to eating too many carbs, it simultaneously sends out inflammation-producing enzymes that attach to collagen, breaking it down and degrading your skin cells. It's this oxidative process (known as *glycation*) that inhibits the effectiveness of collagen (making it stiffer and less flexible), contributing to dull, wrinkled, and saggy skin and triggering specific skin issues, including rosacea and acne.

The other culprit hiding behind the scenes—or underneath your skin—is inflammation. Sugar provokes an inflammatory response that impairs skin cells and, over time, causes a droopy discolored appearance, excess wrinkles, and other signs of premature aging. As you reduce inflammation throughout your body on my program, you'll simultaneously decrease inflammation in your skin and reduce the amount of damage being inflicted unnecessarily on your cells.

However, controlling your ketones isn't the only missing piece to achieving an enviable complexion and reducing (or eliminating) most skin-related issues. Many of the same high-fat, fiber-rich, low-carb foods you'll be eating are packed with essential nutrients that will maintain the strength and integrity of your skin:

- *Artichokes:* Rich in antioxidants and vitamin C, artichokes can improve collagen development and overall skin health. They can also rid your skin of toxins, which will improve skin appearance.

- *Avocados:* Rich in the antioxidant vitamin E, avocados have been shown to reduce skin damage from UV rays[10] and make skin more resilient.[11]

- *Broccoli:* Beyond its many skin-nurturing vitamins and minerals (including vitamin A, vitamin C, and zinc), broccoli is also rich in lutein (a powerful antioxidant proven to filter light and slow down oxidative stress).[12]

- *Dairy, scallops, pumpkin seeds, sesame oil, bacon, darker cuts of poultry, and other zinc-rich fare:* Because of its anti-inflammatory properties, zinc is considered to be one of the leading micronutrients required for regulating your skin and is a powerful mineral used for treating acne,[13] rosacea,[14] and a number of other dermatological disorders.[15]

- *Fatty fish:* Rich in omega-3 fatty acids that reduce inflammation, prevent dry skin,[16] and ward off skin cancer,[17] fatty fish also contain plenty of vitamin E, which may act as a protectant against photoaging (the premature aging of skin caused by UV rays).[18]

- *Leafy greens, eggs, dairy, fish, and other foods high in vitamin A:* Vitamin A stimulates the production of new skin cells and protects you against premature skin aging.[19]

- *Shrimp, beef, sardines, mackerel, salmon, darker cuts of poultry, and other selenium-packed foods:* Selenium preserves skin elasticity and protects your skin from sun damage.[20]

A fiber-dense diet works behind the scenes to improve your skin in other wonderful ways. For example, as Dr. Hoaglin shared, having more fiber in your system slows things down, which in turn gives your body ample time to absorb more nutrients from the food you're eating. So all of those vitamins and minerals I just mentioned are more readily absorbed in greater numbers because of that extra roughage. In addition, fiber's ability to sweep out toxins and waste products from your body is believed to prevent rashes and break-outs,[21] and some experts speculate that certain forms of fiber may help push out pathogens like fungus and yeast before they have a chance to be excreted through your pores.[22]

So how does being "microbially balanced" affect your skin? In addition to improving your immune system to keep your skin healthy,[23] a happy gut can also prevent conditions such as SIBO and dysbiosis, both which have been linked to eczema, rosacea, and other skin situations.[24] It's also believed that specific types of bacteria—such as *Lactobacillus rhamnosus SP1* and *Lactobacillus casei subsp. casei 327*—may be linked to reducing flakiness, improving the skin barrier, and reducing adult acne.[25]

## STRESS AND ANXIETY

Stress is a double-edged sword that's just as good for you as it can be bad for you. You've heard the expression "what doesn't kill you makes you stronger." Well, welcome to stress—to a point.

Healthy stress can be anything that brings your body (or brain) to attention, but gives you enough time to learn, react, and improve. Exercise is one example: push yourself just hard enough so that your muscles know you're serious, and they'll rebuild themselves on a cellular level to be stronger the next time around. Another example is the cellular stress created by autophagy, a process by which your body cannibalizes its own damaged cells. Stressing out your cells by practicing intermittent fasting on a regular basis can make them think they're starved for nutrients and energy, so they begin gobbling up any damaged cells they find lying around—getting rid of damaged proteins and organelles that can promote aging and cause disease.

Then there's the hurtful kind, the bad type that we think of when we say the word *stress*. This is typically chronic stress, the kind that just consistently wears us down and never gives us a chance to get up. My program sets out to minimize by targeting the type of harmful, chronic stress associated with a typical Western diet, and I certainly noticed it started to dissipate once I stepped away from sugar and carbohydrates.

When I was a sugar burner, at times of great stress, I would wake up feeling exhausted and anxious—and remain that way throughout the day. Yet once I utilized fat and ketones, my energy levels stopped dipping, and I found myself more relaxed and in control. I thought it was just me, but when I spoke to other experts, it turns out there were several factors connected to this state of calm. Right now, experts such as Dr. D'Agostino are researching the effects of a ketogenic diet on reducing anxiety, which includes investigating the effects of different formulations of exogenous ketones and MCTs (medium-chain triglycerides). But for the time being, we have made a few connections between keto and tranquility.

For one, even though following a specific diet can be stressful for most people, a ketogenic diet takes some anxiety out of figuring out how you have to eat.[26] This helps reduce stress levels about eating and in your entire life. According to Dr. Volk, most people overlook the flexibility keto gives you since you're no longer eating by the clock. When you're a sugar burner, you experience constant highs and lows in terms of energy, which always leaves you chasing after that next meal to refuel yourself. This perpetual pursuit of energy becomes a stressor we put ourselves under from the time we wake up until the time we go to bed.

But when you're a fat burner, you're no longer desperate to replenish stored glycogen for energy. Instead, your body has the option to run on whatever fats you've just consumed or turn to stored fats for energy—so you're never nervous about that next meal. Once your tummy is no longer at the mercy of time, Volk says a huge portion of stress and anxiety that so many sugar burners possess is off the plate.

The anxious feelings we experience aren't always specifically because of the stressful things that bombard our lives from every direction—they can be because of our fear of not being able to stay on top of everything. When I spoke to Dr. Burke about how a ketogenic diet may act upon this type of stress, she explained that keto can create an improvement loop.

When you're in nutritional ketosis, there's a chance that your cognitive abilities can be better because your brain runs more efficiently on ketones (this is still a growing area of research). Being able to process things much faster and with less brain fog, some amount of your stress and anxiety is reduced. Coincidentally, as you begin to feel less stressed, your cognitive functioning begins to improve. So, which affects the other? It's hard to tell, but regardless, nutritional ketosis still serves as a full circle stress reliever for many. And what is definitely clear is that utilizing ketones and fat instead of sugar may allow you to step back from—and better approach—the things that cause you stress and anxiety, helping you handle those stressors more effectively.

Have you ever wondered if being on a ketogenic diet somehow changes the comfort foods we tend to reach for under stress? As we know all too well, when we feel anxious, many of us crave carbs, which Dr. Burke explained is a natural part of our evolution. Our bodies were meant to survive on fat oxidation for the majority of the time (and go through long periods of fasting) because back in the day, we didn't readily have access to carbohydrates, as most fruit was only seasonally available.

What glycolysis was (and still is) intended for—and what it's still very good at—is giving you instant energy in an emergency. If you're ever in a very stressful, intense situation, your body can quickly use glucose to make adenosine triphosphate (ATP), an energy-storing molecule your muscles rely on to contract, so that you can either fight your way out of a situation or run away.

When you're in that fight-or-flight scenario, Dr. Burke agrees that glucose is best. The problem: When you're stressed, your body often craves sugar and glucose because your brain doesn't know the difference between having to do your taxes and having to run away from a tiger. It simply can't distinguish between the two on a simple physiological level, which is why many people instinctively reach for sugar and high-carb foods to satisfy that need for immediate energy from glucose.

Does this mean that when you become fat adapted and you're under stress, your desire to reach for high-carb foods changes? According to Dr. Burke, if someone is fully keto adapted and experiences a serious physiological stressor, they can't stop glycolysis from happening because it's automatic. A person *might* be more resilient to that stressor, but the research isn't quite there yet in this area.

Infusing fiber into a ketogenic program also minimizes some of the issues that stress can bring on. New research published in the *Journal of Physiology* found that eating high-fiber foods triggers gut bacteria to produce more short-chain fatty acids, which may alleviate certain stress-induced behavioral and physiological alterations that negatively affect gastrointestinal function, metabolism, and immune function.[27]

In fact, a recent study out of the University of Illinois found preclinical evidence that suggests our gut microbiome may contribute to mood and behavior disorders, such as depression, anxiety, and stress.[28] When researchers introduced subjects to certain indigestible compounds to help feed their gut microbiome (specifically fructo-oligosaccharides and galacto-oligosaccharides) and added *Bifidobacteria* into their diet (a good bacteria strain found in fermented foods such as yogurt), it improved anxiety and depression and suppressed biological markers of stress.

Many of the staple foods in my High Fiber Keto program are packed with specific nutrients known to reduce anxiety, such as zinc,[29] omega-3 fatty acids,[30] and B vitamins, as well as such foods as sauerkraut and pickles, which have been shown to possibly lower social anxiety.[31] With the combination of keto, fiber, and a healthy microbiome in one program, you automatically place yourself in a better position to turn down stress or tackle it head on, no matter where or when it may strike.

## HORMONES

They say the eyes are a window to the soul. Similarly, I think hormone levels are a window into your well-being. If you take a look at your hormone snapshot, you'll see it reflects who you are from skin to stress and from head to toe. A growing body of scientific research shows a powerful connection between a ketogenic diet and your hormonal balance. Every part of you reflects your hormonal state.

### Estrogen

Estrogen is a hormone that is most typically associated with sexual and reproductive development in women, though it is involved in virtually every enzymatic system in the body and is a major player in heart health.

When your estrogen levels are low—due to menopause, birth control pills, extreme dieting, or excessive exercising, for example—it diminishes the number of LDL receptors on your liver, making the organ less able to retrieve and eliminate cholesterol.[32]

Therefore many women tend to have higher levels of circulating cholesterol, but it's not the only reason. Estrogen also controls a key enzyme known as *paraoxonase 1 (PON1)*, which helps prevent the oxidation of LDL and significantly reduces your risk of heart disease.[33] If your estrogen is out of balance, the amount of PON1 in your system is reduced, leaving LDL more susceptible to oxidation from free radicals. Once that happens, oxidized LDL can trigger a series of inflammatory responses that can result in atherosclerosis and other serious health issues.

Something that doesn't get enough attention is estrogen's connection to nitric oxide (NO), according to Felice L. Gersh, M.D., OB/GYN, and medical director of the Integrative Medical Group of Irvine, California. Nitric oxide is the magic molecule produced by the endothelium (the lining of your blood vessels) that makes blood vessels expand and increases blood flow.[34]

When you have plenty of nitric oxide, it decreases your risk of clotting and plaque. But when it's in short supply, it causes endothelial dysfunction that can leave you predisposed to hypertension and heart disease.[35] Because estrogen plays a part in inducing nitric oxide production,[36] making sure your hormones are at the proper levels will help to keep your blood vessels happier and healthier.

But that's just the tip of the estrogen iceberg. Estrogen has its hand in virtually every function of the female body. When a woman goes through menopause, she gradually loses this vital hormone produced by her ovaries, which is why it can be exceptionally difficult to ever keep the scales at any point of equilibrium. What make matters worse, as Dr. Gersh stresses, is that we're the only species that tries to manage our reproductive destiny by taking estrogen and progesterone to prevent ovulation.

Today, a large percentage of women are put on birth control pills at some point, despite the fact that we now understand that fertility and metabolic health are inexplicably linked to one another. Meaning, when you knock out fertility, you can't expect everything to go humming along metabolically. Altering the very foundations of our hormones and how they are meant to work rhythmically can cause tremendous metabolic dysfunction to a woman's body, both in the short and long term.

A ketogenic diet can help. As Dr. Gersh explains, anything that lowers chronic inflammation is helpful, which is something a ketogenic diet seems to do.[37] Many people aren't aware that inflammatory cytokines impair ovarian function,[38] but it's been shown that the ovarian follicular fluid of some women with hormonal imbalances has more immune cells that are inflammatory than normal, which keeps ovaries in a perpetually inflamed state and therefore not working properly. But through nutritional ketosis (as well as periodic fasting), you may be able to lower inflammation and restore metabolic homeostasis—something Gersh notes is currently being looked at.

### Testosterone

I had the opportunity to sit down with Dr. Erika Schwartz for a fascinating conversation about hormones and the importance of hormone balance. Dr. Schwartz is an internist, hormone expert, patient advocate, and author who says everyone is looking for a solution to make them look good and feel good. "Everyone is looking for a magic pill. Having your hormones in balance will make you feel good. It's the solution," she says.

Over the years, Dr. Schwartz has treated women of all ages who have suffered from hormonal imbalances and deficiencies that were the cause of a wide variety of health problems. Restoring these patients' hormone balance required looking at their diet, sleep, exercise, and work-life balance.

Along the way, Dr. Schwartz witnessed the positive effects that testosterone can have for women. Testosterone belongs to a class of male hormones known as *androgens*. But it is also produced by women's adrenals and ovaries and is very important in hormonal balance and overall good health.

Dr. Schwartz says testosterone is more important to women's health than most people realize: "Testosterone is a wonderful hormone. Testosterone protects you from heart disease. Testosterone protects you from Alzheimer's and osteoporosis. It helps you think better." Dr. Schwartz also notes, "Women don't realize it's about the hormone balance that having muscle gives you which is health and energy." Testosterone helps to build muscle, which is the best way to protect against osteoporosis.

A study conducted on obese women suffering from PCOS showed that a low-carb diet can reduce testosterone levels in women.[39] Low-carbohydrate diets reduce insulin levels, and anything that reduces insulin will reduce testosterone. I personally experienced a significant decline in my free testosterone level after beginning a keto diet. It's important to make sure you work with your doctor to monitor your hormone levels as you modify your diet.

In contrast, a ketogenic diet improves testosterone levels in men. One 2017 study compared men who ate a keto diet and weight trained with those who ate a traditional Western diet and weight trained. Results showed the men on the keto diet experienced a significant increase in testosterone while the men on the traditional Western diet did not.[40]

In the decade leading up to menopause, many women start to experience symptoms that they may not recognize or realize are being caused by a testosterone imbalance, including sleep problems, anxiety, an inability to juggle responsibilities, brain fog, and bloating. Dr. Schwartz says that if you're with the right doctor, they will ask you questions and not just talk about hormones. The doctor will need to talk about your whole life. Dr. Schwartz believes that unless your doctor listens to you, you won't get the help you need.

### Adiponectin

Adiponectin is involved in glucose and lipid metabolism and acts in the brain to reduce body weight. It is a type of hormone called an *adipokine*, which is released exclusively from your adipose (fat) cells. In a study conducted by the University of Pennsylvania School of Medicine, adiponectin raised the metabolic rate of mice without affecting their appetite.[41] This metabolic increase caused the mice to burn off more heat and lose weight over time and helped to reduce glucose and lipid levels.

Research in humans has shown that adiponectin is an important regulator of insulin sensitivity, glucose and lipid levels, and cardiovascular homeostasis.[42] Researchers say restoring the capacity of adipose tissue to secrete adiponectin has the potential to be an innovative treatment for metabolic diseases.

Getting leaner is one way to optimize your adiponectin level. The more lean your body is, the more adiponectin your fat cells will release. You can maximize your levels by spending more time moving during your day and less time being sedentary.

By replacing carbohydrates with good fats, High Fiber Keto can also help. In a 16-week study of obese, postmenopausal women with type 2 diabetes, those who were given high-linoleic safflower oil significantly increased adiponectin and significantly reduced fasting glucose.[43] These women experienced a reduction in trunk adipose mass (abdominal fat) and an increase in lean mass. I've been passionate about high-linoleic safflower oil for more than 10 years. Even consuming one tablespoon a day can help to transform your belly fat.

## Leptin

Leptin is another adipokine that is produced by your fat cells. But it works differently in your brain than adiponectin by reducing your appetite and making you feel full. When your fat mass increases, your leptin level increases and sends signals to your hypothalamus that you have enough stored fat, which helps to suppress your appetite and prevent overeating until you start to burn some of the stored fat.

Obesity tends to be associated with very high levels of leptin, which implies one would feel full or less hungry and would eat less and lose weight. But obesity causes the leptin system to function improperly through a condition known as *leptin resistance*, where the signal to the brain to stop eating never gets there and the brain continues to think it's starving and drives people to eat and perpetuate the cycle of hunger and weight gain.

Research shows that chronically elevated insulin levels contribute to leptin resistance.[44] You can optimize your leptin levels by avoiding sugar and eating a low-carb diet. Regular exercise and avoiding sedentary behaviors can be beneficial as well.

Another potential cause of leptin resistance is chronic inflammation. Inflammatory foods include foods high in trans fats and sugar. Fatty fish, leafy greens, walnuts, and berries are anti-inflammatory and should be regularly included in your diet.

Research shows the keto diet and other diets rich in fish oil can increase leptin levels in the blood, meaning that delicious fatty fish doubles as an inflammation fighter and a leptin booster![45]

Your leptin levels are affected by how much sleep you get. Insufficient sleep decreases your leptin levels and increases your appetite.[46] This can put you in a vicious cycle of ever-increasing hunger and weight gain. Good sleep is crucial to regulating your leptin level and other hormones that affect your weight.

## Ghrelin

Ghrelin is known as the "hunger hormone" as it is produced in your stomach when your stomach is empty. Ghrelin sends a message to your hypothalamus to tell you to eat. After you eat, your ghrelin level drops. But those who are obese tend to suffer from a ghrelin malfunction. Obesity prevents ghrelin levels from dropping adequately after a meal so the signal to stop eating is weak. Researchers say this can lead to overeating and perpetuate obesity.[47]

Research shows that a keto diet can reduce ghrelin levels. In a study of children with epilepsy, a keto diet significantly reduced ghrelin levels and reduced seizure frequency by more than 50 percent.[48] You can improve ghrelin function by avoiding sugary drinks and foods that contain high-fructose corn syrup. Eating protein can improve satiety and help reduce your ghrelin level after you eat. Intense exercise can also decrease ghrelin levels and offer the added benefit of burning calories and helping build lean mass.

## WATCH THE CLOCK

By now, we know that hormonal balance is crucial to good health. And staying in nutritional ketosis can help.

It turns out that staying in nutritional ketosis also resets your circadian clock, which plays a big part in regulating hormones. The master clock that coordinates the timing of your circadian rhythms, as well as the daily control of hormone secretion, is the suprachiasmatic nucleus (SCN), a tiny region of your brain in your hypothalamus. Dr. Gersh stressed that all hormones run rhythmically, which is why women who work night shifts tend to have reduced fertility, more irregular menstrual cycles, and higher rates of weight gain and metabolic dysfunction.[49]

When you have sufficient quantities of the right hormones, you help to keep your circadian rhythm on track. But if you eat the wrong foods, experience inflammation (which can lead into the brain), or have an estrogen imbalance (which has been shown to have a direct effect on your SCN), it can cause circadian rhythm dysfunction, which is tantamount to metabolic chaos.

According to Dr. Gersh, nutritional ketosis helps reboot your master clock and circadian rhythm, along with other peripheral clocks in your body, which in turn helps reset your metabolic state.

When it comes to hormonal balance, Dr. Schwartz stresses the importance of self-care. She states, "Make sure that what you're doing is for you because if you're okay, your hormones are in balance, you're going to stay young forever, you're going to have energy forever, you're going to be great forever, and you're not going to be hit with a ton of bricks in menopause."

---

As Gersh explained, fiber and a happy microbiome help your hormones in a bidirectional manner. Even though most women associate ovaries with estrogen production, estrogen is also made in significant quantities within Peyer's patches, small masses of lymphoid tissue found within your gut. Estrogen is critical for a healthy functioning gut and immune system; gut-associated lymphoid tissue (GALT) is an essential component of the immune system and the estradiol produced there is immensely important.

You see, there's a portion of your gut microbiome called the *estrobolome*, a collection of microbes capable of metabolizing estrogen by producing *beta-glucuronidase*, an enzyme that helps maintain estrogen homeostasis (or stability).[50] Simply put: Your estrobolome is responsible for recycling estrogen—something especially critical for women in menopause.

But as Gersh stated, when you don't have a healthy microbiome, you end up with either too little or too much beta-glucuronidase, so you stop recycling estrogen as effectively. This is especially critical for pre- and postmenopausal women who need to hold on to as much estrogen as possible. More importantly, it disrupts your estrobolome in a way that impairs estrogen balance and increases your risk of cardiovascular disease,[51] obesity,[52] polycystic ovary syndrome,[53] certain types of cancers (including breast, cervical, and ovarian), metabolic syndrome, and even cognitive dysfunction.[54]

Fibrous foods—and most importantly, according to Gersh, an array of them, because we really don't know yet how every type of food reacts to every type of receptor we possess—work directly with certain estrogen receptor sites in the gut to increase the production of the neurotransmitter serotonin. Serotonin helps to manage your mood, appetite, anxiety, and sleep,[55] so keeping it in abundant supply through the right fiber-rich diet seems like an obvious must. Further to that, serotonin is also the precursor to melatonin, a hormone that makes a big impact on ovarian function.

Melatonin, like all hormones, is a multitasker. And even though most people know it as the sleep hormone—a name it definitely earns by helping to regulate daily body rhythms—it's also one of the most potent antioxidants in the body for reducing inflammation and helping to regulate ovarian function.[56] By fostering a healthy gut through fibrous foods that feed your microbiome, you improve the production of both serotonin and melatonin, helping your ovaries stay as healthy as they can be.

# EMILIE

### *My skin glowed!*

I have tried different diets, but I really wanted to see if I could get into nutritional ketosis and what it was all about.

It wasn't hard, but it did take some time to figure out how to fit it in while keeping my carbs low—and getting the fiber. I felt better when I added some berries and non-starchy vegetables. I learned I *love* to have heavy cream in my coffee, because it keeps me feeling fuller. I also learned that I could eat smaller amounts since the food was so energy-dense.

I'm happy I tried this way of eating. It has opened me up to experimenting with different types of foods that I didn't usually eat. It also forced me to cook at home more and be more thoughtful with my meal planning.

In the end, I got compliments on my complexion, and I feel pretty sure it's because I was eating more healthy fat and less sugar. My skin glowed!

# PART II

# THE STRATEGIES OF HIGH FIBER KETO

## CHAPTER **FIVE**

# THE METABOLIC MENDERS

What if the food you ate could mend your metabolism easily and efficiently, all the while increasing your production of energy-generating ketones? In this chapter you will discover metabolism-mending foods from super herbs to hydrating greens to pre- and probiotics—all of which work with your body's biochemistry to fix a sluggish and inefficient metabolism to give you an optimized metabolism.

We've all had technical hiccups, whether it's with a glitchy phone or a frozen computer. So we all know the first thing that we're supposed to do to see if it will fix the problem: unplug and reboot.

Reset the system, fix the problem, go back to normal.

Our bodies don't have a CTRL+ALT+DEL command or a power cord, but we do have nature's best form of a reboot: a diet that will tell all of your cellular systems to reset, fix themselves, and go back to the way you *should* be.

Just think about all the medical fixes we have today: stitches to close a skin wound, lozenges to soothe a sore throat, antibiotics to trounce enemy invaders, surgery to mend torn tissue or a clogged artery. Yet so often we take for granted that nature's best medicine comes from the food we eat. The right ones are loaded with exactly what you need to heal your body—and help it run as optimally as it can.

This is what High Fiber Keto does:

- Mends your metabolism
- Encourages fat adaptation and nutritional ketosis
- Improves body composition
- Aids in weight management
- Improves production and absorption of ketones and keeps you in nutritional ketosis so you can burn your body fat
- Fights off disease and works toward reversing markers of metabolic syndrome
- Helps you check off your WISH list to feel better and live better every day

Most nutritional programs are built around one goal, and that goal is probably what you would expect—weight loss. But when you're looking for the greatest optimized metabolism possible using a fiber-rich, nutritionally balanced ketogenic diet, it takes an intricately designed program. It takes a diet plan that provides enough fiber, along with other prebiotic and probiotic foods that feed the microbiome and immune system, all while working toward a state of nutritional ketosis.

A fiber-rich, nutritionally balanced ketogenic diet can satisfy these goals plus weight loss simultaneously.

Unlike other ketogenic programs that mostly rely on a random mix of high-fat, moderate-protein, and low-carb foods to encourage fat adaptation and ketone production, my program integrates an exact blend of specific nutrients that simultaneously support nutritional ketosis, promote metabolic health, fuel you with fiber, and nurture your microbiome. Because of this specific formula, High Fiber Keto allows you to eat a wider variety of foods—and experience a greater range of flavors and tastes—than you might expect, all while optimizing your health!

And yes, it all tastes deliciously good as well.

Whole grains, legumes, and starchy fruits and veggies may be rich in fiber and nutrients, but for most of us they contribute to weight gain, inflammation, and a whole host of health problems for those already at a metabolic disadvantage.

My plan is designed to help you minimize consumption of these metabolically disadvantaging foods and focus on the foods—in the right ratio—to help you optimize your metabolism. Using the specific combination of foods I've laid out in your meal plan, you'll get on the right path.

These foods—if you consume them in the right combination—will do exactly what you hope they will: help you reset your body and work with your body's biochemistry to give you an optimized metabolism.

Let's dive in to the specific foods you'll be enjoying on High Fiber Keto and their benefits for your health and total body wellness. I like to call them the *metabolic menders*.

## MCTS

It's not a coincidence that MCTs (medium-chain triglycerides) are the first metabolic mender on the list. MCTs are the nutritional headliner because of their incredible power and effect on your body.

MCTs can take a ketogenic diet to the next level by boosting ketones in circulation, providing an alternative fuel to glucose for energy, and curbing your carb and sugar cravings. That's why my specifically designed meal plan is rich in nourishing fatty acid sources packed with this metabolic mender.

Fatty acids (the building blocks of lipids or fats) are made up of atoms that range in length. Most fats contain long-chain fatty acids (at least 14 carbon atoms long), but some forms of fat contain medium-chain fatty acids (between 6 and 12 carbon atoms long).

What makes MCTs so special is how they are absorbed and metabolized. Because of their shorter fatty-acid chain length, MCTs go straight to the liver. This differs from the path for dietary carbohydrates and protein, which are broken down throughout the digestive system and then sent to the liver for processing and delivery to appropriate tissues through a slower process.

Traditional dietary fats also take a longer route to becoming energy for your body. These fats travel through the digestive system, and then head to the lymphatic system before finally making it to the liver.

Translation: MCTs break down much faster, allowing medium-chain fatty acids to be metabolized and used for energy immediately. This difference (among others) leads to higher ketone production because fat is being metabolized more quickly.

## GREENS THAT PRODUCE RESULTS

Metabolism is a gift that keeps on giving when you have a diet that includes cruciferous vegetables, artichokes, leafy greens, and other veggies. That's not to say that all vegetables are created equal. For the most part, vegetables grown above the soil (think lettuce, cauliflower, and broccoli) are typically lower in carbohydrates than those grown below, such as root vegetables like sweet potatoes and carrots. But that doesn't mean there isn't plenty of variety you can eat without having to worry about slipping out of nutritional ketosis.

When you're eating with an optimized metabolism in mind, selecting specific fiber-dense, microbiome-beneficial veggies allows you to create the perfect blend of vitamins, minerals, enzymes, and phytonutrients that encourages nutritional ketosis and supports metabolic health. That's why for 22 days you'll be eating meals and snacks built around the incredible edibles below.

### Hydrating Veggies

What science has shown us is that you can't truly hydrate the body through water alone.[1] The key is to eat the types of foods that allow your body to bring water more directly into your cells.

Dana Cohen, M.D., the author of *Quench*, shared with me the exciting science around how our bodies store water and the effect of "gel" or "structured" water, the liquid with an extra hydrogen and oxygen atom found in plant and animal cells. So instead of $H_2O$, it's actually $H_3O_2$. It contains a higher concentration of nutrients, including glucose and sodium, which are thought to make it more hydrating—easier for your body to absorb and retain water more efficiently.

Before your body transitions to fat-adaptation, it will turn to glucose as a form of energy first. Since you are not consuming the same level of total carbohydrates, your body will break down stored glucose in the form of *glycogen* before turning to fat. The glycogen molecule has a water molecule in its structure, so when you break down glycogen, you also release water in the process. This is a normal process that happens any time you break down glycogen, but during the initial stages of fat adaptation, it happens at a more noticeable rate.

At first you may lose some "water weight" on a high-fat plan, which is why it is so important to stay well hydrated at all times, but you should pay especially close attention during the first few days and weeks of carbohydrate restriction. Hydrate routinely, ensure proper electrolyte balance, and fill your plate with ample hydrating vegetables that are at least 70 percent water—foods such as broccoli, spinach, celery, cucumber, cabbage, mushrooms, and lettuce. These types of veggies are filled with gel water that may help make it easier to stay hydrated. In addition, drinking bone broth, adding chia seeds to smoothies and salads, and cooking with flaked, unsweetened coconut and coconut oil can add more structured water to your diet in an easy daily way.

In addition to quenching your thirst, some of the water-rich veggies in my program come with metabolic extras:

*Broccoli:* Besides being one of the best foods to eat for reducing your risk of cardiovascular disease,[2] this cruciferous vegetable is loaded with sulforaphane, a potent phytochemical that reduces oxidative stress,[3] combats inflammation,[4] and helps fight cancer.[5]

*Cauliflower:* Fiber friendly and high in choline (a nutrient that helps support metabolism and prevents cholesterol from building up in the liver[7]), cauliflower boasts one of the highest saturations of glucosinolates, a natural compound that detoxifies and may help in cancer prevention, of any vegetable.[8]

*Celery:* Not only is celery a great source of fiber, it is bursting with water and electrolytes (mainly sodium) to help keep you hydrated. It has anti-inflammatory properties that can aid in maintaining proper blood pressure and cholesterol levels.[6]

*Collard leaves:* This often-ignored leafy green veggie is overflowing with nutrients, including vitamin K to keep your bones strong, vitamin A for your immune system, and a host of cancer-fighting glucosinolates.

*Cucumbers:* Cucumbers are a low-calorie, powerful vegetable with detoxing and antiaging properties. They are great for weight loss while providing off-the-charts water content and good amounts of sodium, potassium, magnesium, and vitamins K and C.

*Spinach:* High in vitamin K, magnesium, and insoluble fiber, this leafy legend is also abundant in nitrates that help lower blood pressure and reduce your risk of cardiovascular disease.[9]

*Yellow squash:* Loaded with carotenoids (which lower blood pressure and reduce inflammation) and manganese (a mineral that helps the body process fats and carbohydrates and may reduce PMS symptoms),[10] a daily serving may reduce your risk of heart disease by 23 percent.[11]

*Zucchini:* This low-carb, high-water veggie has tremendous antioxidative properties[12] and contains both soluble and insoluble fiber to nourish your gut and boost your insulin sensitivity.[13]

### Less Water-Based, but Equally Wonderful

While some greens may have less water in comparison to others, they still offer an array of gut-sustaining bacteria and nutrients, along with a host of other unbelievable metabolic benefits.

*Arugula:* Besides its cancer-quelling abilities,[14] this peppery green is fortified with folate, magnesium, and potassium, which collectively support cardiovascular health.

*Dandelion leaves:* Full of nutrients, including magnesium and potassium that help control blood pressure, this prebiotic weed also contains chicoric and chlorogenic acid, two compounds that may lower blood sugar and have other antidiabetic properties.[15]

*Endive and kale:* Both endive and kale contain quercetin, a polyphenolic flavonoid that reduces blood pressure,[16] and kaempferol, a flavonoid shown to have a wide range of anti-inflammatory, antimicrobial, anticancer, cardioprotective, neuroprotective, antidiabetic, anti-osteoporotic, and antiallergic benefits.[17]

*Garlic:* This prebiotic supports your immune system in fighting off cancer, though its strongest asset may be allicin, a compound shown to have myriad healthy effects, from lowering cholesterol and blood pressure to inhibiting bad bacteria and fungi.[18]

*Jicama:* Besides being a powerful prebiotic, this root veggie is full of LDL-lowering fiber that keeps your blood sugar steady, and it contains plenty of heart-healthy antioxidants, including vitamin C, vitamin E, and selenium.

*Seaweed:* In addition to being a prebiotic, seaweed contains fucoxanthin, a carotenoid that may have anti-obesity effects by impacting blood sugar levels[19] and helping to metabolize fat.[20]

## SUPER HERBS

Super herbs are culinary herbs and spices with medicinal properties that allow us to use food as medicine for metabolic healing. Often skipped in everyday American cooking, super herbs are an integral part of my High Fiber Keto meal plan and, along with fiber, I consider them to be my essential ingredients for keto success. The spices and herbs you'll be using during the 22 days of the plan will boost the flavor of every meal and snack without knocking you out of nutritional ketosis, and while offering additional unique health benefits. Herbs and spices are one of the best ways to boost beneficial plant compounds, such as polyphenols and carotenoids, along with vitamins and minerals. These compounds can act as antioxidants to protect your cells from toxins and free radical damage. The result: Being better equipped to manage inflammation and a better-functioning metabolism.

The super herbs I've selected to complement and enhance your High Fiber Keto diet plan provide blood sugar support, improve digestion, increase detoxification, boost cardiovascular health, and more. Herbs are also a source of antimicrobial compounds that help to protect your digestive system and body from food-borne pathogens. Simply by adding 1 to 2 tablespoons of fresh or 1 to 2 teaspoons of dried thyme or rosemary as a rub or marinade for meat, you can help prevent the formation of compounds like heterocyclic amines, which damage DNA and have been linked to cancer.[21]

Here are just a few ingredients that your appetite will appreciate and that will magnify your metabolism and heal you from within:

*Basil:* This natural anti-inflammatory[22] is rich in vitamin A, vitamin K, potassium, and calcium and has also been shown to have antibacterial properties,[23] helping to restrict the growth of numerous bad strains of bacteria.

*Cacao powder and cacao nibs:* Besides being delicious in their own right, both cacao powder and cacao nibs contain polyphenols and serve as prebiotics that increase the population of beneficial bacteria in your gut.[24]

*Cardamom:* Powerful in taste, this fiery-sweet spice has been shown to lower blood pressure,[25] defend against bad bacteria,[26] and potentially fight cancer.[27]

*Ceylon cinnamon:* Ceylon cinnamon is considered "true cinnamon" and is of the highest quality. Loaded with metabolism-supportive antioxidants such as calcium, iron, and manganese, cinnamon has been shown to reduce inflammation,[28] have beneficial effects on all five factors associated with metabolic syndrome (especially insulin sensitivity, blood pressure, and body weight), and possibly be vital to preventing type 2 diabetes and cardiovascular-related diseases.[29]

*Cilantro:* Packed with vitamins A, C, and K and phytonu-trients such as the NAD+-boosting apigenin and luteolin, along with geraniol, limonene, and quercetin, cilantro has a long history of culinary and medicinal use. It has been known to chelate, or bind to, heavy metals in the body, thus supporting detoxification pathways and reducing oxidative stress.

*Curry powder:* This bountiful blend can consist of many things besides curry leaves, including turmeric, cinnamon, cardamom, cloves, nutmeg, bay leaves, and other spices. It offers a rich assortment of antioxidants, including curcumin (a main component of turmeric, which is an ingredient in curry powder), which has been shown to help kill a wide variety of tumor cells[30] and aid with digestion.[31]

*Ginger:* Besides being a great nausea reliever,[32] this anti-oxidant may decrease your risk of cancer,[33] promote the growth of beneficial bacteria in the gut,[34] and have a ma-jor impact on glucose control, insulin sensitivity, and the improvement of your blood lipid profile.[35]

*Oregano:* This common spice is far from ordinary when it comes to your metabolic health, containing compounds that kill bad bacteria[36] and serve as potent antioxidant, anti-inflammatory, antidiabetic, and cancer suppressor agents.[37]

*Red pepper flakes:* The active component in this spice is capsaicin, which may have beneficial effects on metabolic syndrome[38] by increasing fat oxidation, improving insulin sensitivity, decreasing body fat, and improving heart and liver function.[39]

*Rosemary leaves:* This fragrant form of mint is believed to have anti-inflammatory, antidiabetic, and anticancer properties[40] and may potentially suppress tumors in the colon, breast, liver, and stomach, as well as melanoma and leukemia cells.[41]

*Thyme:* In addition to plenty of vitamins and minerals, thyme contains the naturally occurring compound thymol, a strong antimicrobial antioxidant, an anticarcinogen that may inhibit cancer development, and an anti-inflammatory.[42]

*Turmeric:* Known for lowering inflammation, this pungent spice has also been linked to reversing insulin resistance, hyperglycemia, hyperlipidemia, and other symptoms related to obesity.[43]

## FRIENDLY FIBER

Not all types of fiber-rich fare work in step with a ketogenic program. But as I've described, the high-fiber, minimal-carb sources you'll be counting on in the High Fiber Keto plan will keep the ketones coming. Even better, you'll be eating an incredible variety of contrasting, plant-based fiber sources that will really build out your microbiome.

As you've learned, both soluble and insoluble fibers are important for digestive health, which is why I've emphasized many sources of fiber-rich foods, from prebiotics to everything in between.

These are some of the top stars to look out for in my program:

*Artichoke hearts:* Part of the thistle family, artichokes are rich in soluble fiber, particularly inulin,[44] and can act as a prebiotic to improve the microbiome;[45] provide key nutrients, including the electrolyte minerals sodium, potassium, and magnesium;[46] and protect and improve the health of the liver.[47] Shown to raise good cholesterol and lower both bad cholesterol and triglycerides,[48] artichoke hearts contain luteolin, an antioxidant that specifically inhibits intestinal cholesterol absorption.[49]

*Avocado:* This fibrous, high-fat fruit lowers LDL, raises HDL, and reduces triglycerides. In fact, regular avocado consumption may make you 50 percent less likely to develop metabolic syndrome.[50]

*Berries:* All berries offer plenty of fiber, and you'll be mixing and matching them to support as many different microbial species and experience as many phytonutrients and antioxidants as possible. Each type of berry features different polyphenols, such as anthocyanins in blueberries, which may improve cardiovascular health,[51] and ellagic acid in raspberries, a phenol that may bind to certain chemicals responsible for cancer.[52]

*Chia seeds:* Packed with omega-3 fatty acids and able to absorb up to 12 times their weight in water, leaving you feeling more satiated, chia seeds have been shown to aid in blood pressure regulation[53] and keep blood sugar levels stable.[54] High in soluble fiber, these seeds are fermentable by the bacteria in your microbiome and effectively bulk the stool to support digestion and healthy bowel habits.

*Flaxseed:* This tiny seed is an anticancer agent[55] and is equally impressive at regulating blood sugar, lowering LDL cholesterol, and decreasing blood pressure.[56] It contains the omega-3 fatty acid alpha-linolenic acid, which is anti-inflammatory, and lignans, which promote estrogen balance.

*Hemp seeds:* These nutrient dense nuts (that's right—they're not technically a seed) are loaded with the amino acid arginine, which in turn produces nitric oxide, the vital neurotransmitter used for a variety of heart-healthy functions, including helping blood vessels relax, lowering inflammation, and fighting off bad bacteria.

But these aren't the only sources of fiber. Here is how much of the nutrient is in many of the other metabolic menders in this chapter:

| Food | Portion | Fiber | Food | Portion | Fiber |
|------|---------|-------|------|---------|-------|
| Almonds | 1 ounce | 4 g | Peanuts | 1 ounce | 2 g |
| Asparagus, cooked | 1 cup | 4 g | Pepper (green or yellow) | 1 medium | 2 g |
| Artichokes | 1 large | 10.4 g | Pumpkin | 1 cup | 0.6 g |
| Arugula | 1 cup | 0.4 g | Radicchio | 1 leaf | 0.1 g |
| Avocado, raw | ½ fruit | 9 g | Raspberries | 1 cup | 8 g |
| Blackberries, raw | 1 cup | 8 g | Red cabbage, cooked | 1 cup | 4 g |
| Blueberries, raw | 1 cup | 4 g | Sauerkraut | 2 tbsp | 1 g |
| Broccoli, cooked | 1 cup | 5 g | Sesame seeds | ¼ cup | 4 g |
| Brussels sprouts, cooked | 1 cup | 6 g | Spaghetti squash, cooked | 1 cup | 2 g |
| Cauliflower, cooked | 1 cup | 5 g | Spinach, cooked | 1 cup | 4 g |
| Chia seeds | 1 ounce | 9–10 g | Strawberries, raw | 1 cup | 3 g |
| Coconut, shredded | 1 cup | 7 g | Sunflower seeds | ¼ cup | 3 g |
| Collard greens, boiled | 1 cup | 8 g | Swiss chard, cooked | 1 cup | 4 g |
| Endive (chopped) | 1 cup | 1.5 g | Walnuts | 1 ounce | 2 g |
| Flaxseed | 1 ounce | 8 g | Watercress | 10 sprigs | 0.1 g |
| Green beans | 1 cup | 3 g | Yellow squash, cooked | 1 cup | 1.2 g |
| Hemp seeds | 3 tbsp | 1.2 g | Zucchini, cooked | 1 cup | 3 g |
| Jicama, raw | 1 cup | 6 g | | | |
| Kale, cooked | 1 cup | 3 g | | | |

# THE NIMBLEST NUTS AND SMARTEST SEEDS

Just because nuts and seeds are both high fat doesn't necessarily mean every single variety should be on your metabolic menu. Pistachios, chestnuts, and cashews, for example, are high-carb choices that can affect your ability to reach nutritional ketosis. That's why you'll be utilizing an assortment of low-carb, fiber-rich nuts and seeds and enjoying modest amounts of certain versions that may be slightly higher in carbohydrates.

*Almonds:* The health benefits of this low-carb high-antioxidant ally are endless, which is why you'll be eating this nut in the form of almond flour and almond meal and just enjoying them whole! In addition to their ability to reduce oxidative damage[57] and help build stronger bones,[58] almonds have been shown to raise HDL levels and make circulating HDLs more efficient at transporting cholesterol from tissues to your liver so that it's processed by your body faster.[59]

*Macadamia and pine nuts:* Tree nuts have been shown to decrease triglycerides and fasting blood glucose,[60] as well as potentially impact the gut microbiome in a way that affects body composition and prevents weight gain.[61]

*Pecans and pecan butter:* This often-underappreciated nut has been shown to double gamma-tocopherol (vitamin E) levels in the body and decrease unhealthy oxidation of LDL cholesterol in the blood by as much as 33 percent.[62]

*Pili nuts:* These are a wonderful source of fiber and contain more magnesium than any other nut. They reduce inflammation, lower cholesterol levels, aid in weight loss, and boost immunity.

*Pumpkin seeds (pepitas):* Fortified with omega-3 fatty acids, pumpkin seeds help to keep your heart and blood vessels healthy, aid in elevating HDL levels, and may even be beneficial in minimizing menopause symptoms.[63]

*Sunflower seeds:* High in heart-healthy vitamin E and copper, as well as the antioxidant selenium (which protects your body against cell damage), these tiny titans have been shown to lower certain metabolic markers, including blood glucose, cholesterol, and blood pressure.[64]

*Walnuts:* One of the best nuts for improving cardio, metabolic, and gastrointestinal health,[65] walnuts are ideal for increasing the number of butyrate-producing microbes in your gut.[66]

## BIOME-BENEFICIAL NUTRIENTS

Keeping your gut happy, healthy, and helping to produce ketones takes the right fusion of prebiotics and probiotics. Here are just a few of the foods and ingredients that will keep your gut glowing and your heart and health humming.

*Apple cider vinegar (raw):* Brimming with good bacteria and enzymes essential for a healthy microbiome, apple cider vinegar reduces belly fat and triglycerides,[67] lowers blood sugar,[68] and targets and kills bad bacteria, including *E. coli, staphylococcus aureus*, and *candida albicans*.[69]

*Cabbage:* This anti-inflammatory vegetable (including in the form of sauerkraut)[70] contains plenty of insoluble fiber for good bacteria to feast on, along with soluble fiber and the plant compound phytosterol, which team up to block the absorption of cholesterol and lower your LDL levels.[71]

*Fermented pickles:* In addition to their probiotic power, fermented pickles are rich in vitamin K (essential for blood clotting) and have a high sodium content (needed for kidney excretion while in nutritional ketosis).

*Greek yogurt, yogurt, and coconut yogurt:* High in probiotics, these yogurts are metabolic heroes since they have been linked with lower levels of circulating triglycerides, glucose, and lower systolic blood pressure and insulin resistance.[72]

*Kefir:* This fermented star contains a host of probiotics and nutrients, is high in protein and calcium (contributing to bone health and lowering the risk of osteoporosis), is low in calories, and has antibacterial properties.

*Prebiotic veggies:* Prebiotic veggies, including dandelion greens, jicama, leeks, and onions, are plentiful with inulin, a soluble fiber that's been shown to restore the gut microbiome and prevent bacteria from invading epithelial cells within the intestine.[73]

## MINERAL-RICH SEAFOOD

Naturally low in carbohydrates and high in omega-3 fatty acids, fish and shellfish are ideal for a ketogenic diet. Choosing the ones in sync with your metabolic goals, however, is another story. My program includes the finest fatty seafood that works with your healthful ambitions and is naturally lower in mercury and other environmental toxins.

*Anchovies:* Sometimes used as a cauliflower pizza topping, this fish provides a bevy of nutrients (including folate, calcium, magnesium, and vitamins E and K). Also rich in vitamin A, anchovies help prevent macular degeneration and boost eye health.

*Sardines:* These may be small, but they contain ample amounts of omega-3s, including EPA and DHA fatty acids, which may have a positive effect on hyperglycemia, insulin resistance, hyperlipidemia, and inflammation.[74]

*Sea scallops:* Brimming with magnesium and potassium to keep your heart healthy, sea scallops are also an excellent source of zinc, a mineral that works with more than 300 enzymes within your body[75] and assists in a variety of important tasks, including protein synthesis, wound healing, and cell division.

*Shrimp:* Consider shrimp to be your circulatory system's best friend, from the way they improve your ratio of LDL to HDL cholesterol and lower triglycerides.[76] They are also an incredible source of iodine, a mineral vital for thyroid health that many are deficient in.

*Wild Alaskan cod:* This flaky fish is full of good-for-you nutrients, including $B_{12}$, a vitamin essential for forming red blood cells,[77] and phosphorus, a mineral critical to the health of your heart, making new cells, and teaming up with certain B vitamins to give you cellular energy.

*Wild Alaskan salmon:* With nearly negligible carbs and an abundance of B vitamins, potassium, and selenium, this strong swimmer contains astaxanthin, a compound shown to reduce LDL cholesterol and boost HDL cholesterol.[78]

*Wild mackerel:* This oily fish contains B-complex vitamins, selenium, magnesium, and potassium. One fillet of wild mackerel provides more than the recommended daily allowance of vitamin D, which has been shown to help lower your risk of coronary heart disease[79] and heart failure.[80]

## OVERACHIEVING OILS

You'll be cooking with and mixing in different types of oil that will work in tandem with your optimized metabolism. Most contain our favorite MCTs, whose smaller size allows them to get shuttled straight to your liver, where they are burned for bountiful energy and trigger an increase in ketone body production. But in the interest of an optimized metabolism, we'll focus on the oils that can help keep your health under control in conjunction with nutritional ketosis. These are some of my favorites that you'll be counting on for more than just ketones.

*Avocado oil:* This antioxidant-rich oil is revered for improving cardiovascular health, weight management, and blood glucose control,[81] and it's overflowing in oleic acid, a monounsaturated omega-9 fatty acid shown to reduce inflammation[82] and lower your risk of breast cancer.[83]

*Coconut oil:* The high lauric acid content in coconut oil makes it a strong antimicrobial agent.[84] Plus, it's been shown to positively impact several factors of metabolic syndrome, including raising HDL cholesterol and decreasing waist circumference.[85] Choose an oil that's pure, cold-pressed, and non-GMO to ensure that it's been extracted and purified using enzymes and not chemicals.

*MCT oil:* This one is pretty self-explanatory, right? Select a high-quality, organic or whole-food version since about 80 percent of MCT oils are conventionally grown and processed and could have traces of toxins, mold, or heavy metals due to chemical (hexane) extraction or lack of safety testing.

*Olive oil:* This healthy oil has been shown to significantly reduce your risk of all-cause mortality, cardiovascular disease, and strokes,[86] and contains the antioxidant oleocanthal, an anti-inflammatory proven to be as strong as ibuprofen.[87]

*Sesame oil:* Rich in monounsaturated and polyunsaturated fats and plenty of cardio-friendly nutrients such as zinc and vitamins B and E, this nutty oil is known for significantly improving cholesterol levels and lowering blood pressure.[88]

*Tea-seed oil:* This oil is a polyphenol powerhouse and contains high levels of vitamin E, an antioxidant which prevents rancidity during storage and thus prolongs shelf life.[89] It is composed of almost 90 percent unsaturated fat, linking it to lower LDL cholesterol and harmful triglyceride levels in the body. The 485 degrees Fahrenheit smoke point is higher than most traditional cooking oils, making it ideal for a variety of cooking applications.

## DECADENT DAIRY

For those of you who consume dairy, choosing products without excess sugar and carbs that could bump you out of nutritional ketosis is one concern. Being cautious about not accidentally raising the amount of protein you're eating each day is another, since many dairy products contain ample amounts of fat alongside protein. The good news is that I have taken these issues into consideration, which is why this program includes specific types of cheeses, creams, milks, and butter that ignite metabolic healing and still encourage fat adaptation.

Quality is key when it comes to animal products. Look for organic and pasture-raised options as much as possible. Not only will you consume fewer hormones and antibiotics with these versions, but you'll also get more nutrition from higher levels of fat-soluble nutrients such as vitamin D, vitamin A, and carotenoids.

As you shop for each type of cheese, consider buying the smallest size possible, even if you have to buy several pieces to have enough to make the recipes, and then buy different brands of the same cheese made in different parts of the world. Every form of cheese has its own unique microbe community, and the fungi and other bacteria found in cheese change depending on its place of origin.[90] And as you now know, variety is important!

> *Goat cheese:* Low carb, deliciously creamy, and teeming with a vast array of probiotics,[91] particularly *Lactobacillus plantarum 564*, goat cheese has been shown to be more filling and a better appetite suppressor than conventional dairy from cow's milk, which has undergone more pro-cessing, removing valuable nutrients and adding unneces-sary toxins, such as hormones and antibiotics. And while some dairy contains casein, products made from goat's and sheep's milk contain a higher amount of a specific type called *A2 casein*, which may be less inflammatory and more easily digested than cow's dairy.[92]

> *Grass-fed butter:* Abundant in saturated fats and butyrate, grass-fed butter contains plenty of omega-3 fatty acids, particularly CLA (conjugated linoleic acid), a natural form of trans fats that may regulate insulin,[93] protect against obesity,[94] and possibly prevent atherosclerosis.[95]

> *Various other cheeses (including cheddar, blue cheese, feta, Gouda, mozzarella, and Parmesan):* Cheese significantly

increases butyrate production, while simultaneously decreasing TMAO, a metabolite produced by gut bacteria that, when present in abundance, significantly increases your risk of cardiovascular disease.[96] Cheese helps lower cholesterol via bile soaps during digestion.[97]

## EGGCEPTIONAL EGGS

Eggs are the perfect food for your keto diet because they are considered to be in the top three highest-quality proteins, are a great source of fat, and pack the punch of containing almost every nutrient that your body needs. I often think of the egg yolk as nature's multivitamin. Eggs from chickens raised on pasture are going to be even more nutrient-dense.

Although bursting with nutrients, including vitamin D and choline (which supports both metabolism and liver function), the egg sometimes gets a bad rap due to its abundance of dietary cholesterol. To clarify, the cholesterol in foods is not the same as that which is in the blood, and foods that contain cholesterol typically don't have an effect on blood cholesterol levels. In fact, studies indicate that their consumption doesn't affect your risk of cardiovascular disease.[98] A recent study found that subjects who ate at least a dozen eggs weekly for three months never experienced an increase in cardiometabolic risk factors.[99] The most recent government nutrition guidelines have even removed the recommendation to limit dietary cholesterol.[100]

## SMART SWEETENERS

A very interesting and much-debated issue among keto diet experts and enthusiasts is the place that keto-approved sweeteners have and whether they are helpful or harmful. One of my hopes for you as you embark on your High Fiber Keto journey is that your tastes will slowly but surely shift. Over time, you'll find that you rely less on sweetness, and that constant desire for dessert will naturally diminish. With that said, we all want a delicious keto treat once in a while, and some sweeteners are definitely healthier and less damaging than others.

Keep in mind that all sweet tastes will induce an insulin response in the body, which can perpetuate cravings for sugars and carbohydrates. Be mindful and conscious of whether or not sugar cravings are a big challenge for you and take the following sweetener suggestions with a grain of (sugary) salt! Strive to use them in moderation.

*Monk fruit:* Pure monk-fruit sweetener has come onto the scene of noncaloric sweeteners recently and is personally one of my favorite ways to sweeten the occasional keto treat. Compounds in monk fruit have antioxidant activity, and animal studies have found it to lower blood sugar,[101] mitigate oxidative stress,[102] and improve blood lipids.[103] The main downside of a high-quality monk fruit is that it tends to be the priciest of the keto sweeteners.

*Stevia:* Native to South America, stevia has been used both as a sweetener and medicinally for centuries. The two primary compounds in stevia that provide its sweet taste are rebaudioside A and stevioside, the compound that is responsible for many of stevia's health benefits, including lowered blood pressure and blood sugar levels.[104]

*Erythritol:* Sugar alcohols like erythritol have become very popular on the keto scene and are increasingly used in many food products. Erythritol seems to have far less potential for digestive upset than other sugar alcohols and is likely tolerated well in small amounts by most people.[105] It is 60 to 70 percent as sweet as table sugar and tastes fairly similar to sugar without the unpleasant aftertaste that some find with stevia. Sugar alcohols also seem to have a fairly neutral effect on blood sugar and insulin levels.[106]

All in all, use these smart sweeteners for a once-in-a-while indulgence instead of depending on them to satisfy a sweet tooth that you'll likely find to be a distant memory quite soon.

## CAN'T-MISS MEATS

To stay in nutritional ketosis, you will need to turn to specific fat-dense meats and poultry rather than leaner options, but not every high-fat meat is on the metabolic menu. You'll also be choosing grass-fed options, which are higher in antioxidants and omega-3 fats than grain-fed meats.[107] Here are some of the choices that will give you a greater metabolic edge.

> *Bacon (nitrite- and nitrate-free) and pasture-raised pork:* The "other white meat" has plenty of nutrients, including selenium, zinc, $B_{12}$, phosphorus, and especially taurine, an important amino acid that's been shown to help lower your risk of coronary heart disease.[108]
>
> *Darker/fattier forms of chicken:* Bone-in, skin-on chicken breasts, skin-on thighs, and wings contain more iron, selenium, and zinc than leaner cuts. Chicken in general is an excellent source of niacin, a form of vitamin $B_3$ that aids in lipid control and helps prevent diseases of the heart and blood vessels.[109]
>
> *Lamb:* Rich in both saturated and monounsaturated fats, lamb is also extremely high in conjugated linoleic acid (CLA), taurine, and iron, which may have a protective effect against coronary artery disease.[110]
>
> *Turkey:* This bird offers plenty of heart-helping nutrients, including potassium, selenium, B vitamins, and niacin. It's also a great source of the amino acid tryptophan, which has been shown to improve both mood and sleep quality.[111]

As you prepare to start my 22-day plan, you will see how I use these foods to help you get into nutritional ketosis—and provide you with a balance of nutrients to help you sustain energy, fight off disease, and *feel* better.

Above all, I want you to see that the High Fiber Keto diet is not just about getting you into nutritional ketosis, but also about making sure that your diet has the best ingredients that can help your over-all well-being. By following my plan, you'll be able to maximize this nutritionally powerful diet to help steer your metabolism in the right direction by using fuel more efficiently and to improving your body composition. As you begin, you will want to know how to get additional support because for many people this can be a very big change. And that is what we will look into next.

## BRANDI

### *I was able to lose weight—and I felt more motivated!*

Once I hit my mid-30s, I really noticed what so many women feel. Everything started to slow down, and I began to struggle with my weight. My weight went up and down with every new diet I tried. I'd lose pounds—and then put them right back on. With a few bonus pounds too.

I tried writing it off as a slow metabolism—that's what I told my friends and family anyway. And I just chalked it up to what happens with age. My new normal, right?

But my joints hurt, too, and I knew that was because I was carrying too much extra weight and the fact that I had dropped exercise and movement from my life. My mood was horrible, and I had no desire—zero—to do anything.

After I started High Fiber Keto, I was energized. I was healthier. I was motivated. The combination of veggies, herbs, seafood, dairy, and meat options worked with my body instead of against it. I was actually shocked at what I was experiencing. And I lost seven pounds in the first two weeks and 30 pounds all together. And I've kept it off! That's something I've never done before.

For years, I thought I knew what worked for me and I made the "slow metabolism" excuse over and over. Neither was true. So don't be afraid to step out of your comfort zone and try something new. The results may just surprise you.

CHAPTER **SIX**

# SIX TO STRENGTHEN

## How to Optimize Your Diet and Gain the Ultimate Metabolism

Fun story: For my first book, *Glow15*, I considered many titles. (The book was centered around the science of autophagy, but that doesn't really have a nice ring to it!) Of all the options that my team discussed, one of the leading contenders was *Boost*.

For a long time, I loved *Boost* as a title, because I connected with what it meant on many levels—mostly because the word has a turbocharged feel to it and a meaning that speaks to so many important points in the health arena. Namely, what can you do to get an extra advantage? What can you do to take your foundational program and give it an extra kick? What can you do to go from *survive* to *thrive*?

After all, a boost is like adding a hot spice to a recipe, extra credit to an exam, or more memory to a computer.

It's a bonus, and it improves your outcome.

That's the way I think about certain nutrients and supplements: they can boost your overall nutrition and health because they can

(1) fill in the gaps left by things that might be missing, and (2) give you a cellular supercharge.

As someone who has been involved in the health and wellness field for much of my life and my entire career, I've experienced first-hand how even when you follow the most regimented food plan, it's rarely possible to obtain every single nutrient our bodies need every single day. On top of that, so many other factors can create nutritional deficiencies in our diet.

For example, due to modern food production and filtration systems, the water and soil used to produce our foods contain fewer nutrients, a deficit that is passed on to what we grow or raise. It's also understood that due to the use of pesticides, fruits and vegetables don't have to work as hard to defend themselves to survive, which makes them less dense in certain nutrients that can improve our health. In addition, our ability to absorb nutrients declines with age as breaking down food gradually becomes more difficult for our bodies.

Even though I believe getting nutrients directly from food should always be your main focus, relying on food alone can potentially leave you nutritionally imbalanced, putting you at a metabolic disadvantage. That's why I am equally passionate about using nutritional supplementation to fill in any gaps, particularly when it comes to five crucial nutrient groups—five areas that the scientific experts I've worked with consider indispensable when following a fiber-rich, biome-building, ketogenic diet to optimize your metabolism.

I am the founder of a whole-body wellness and healthy-living lifestyle company that offers functional food, nutrients, and beauty products at NaomiWhittel.com. I have developed more than 130 award-winning supplements throughout my career in health and wellness, and—with my team of researchers, farmers, and growers—have personally co-created a series of products that work best with this program, which you can find more information about in the Resources section.

It is important that you take advantage of the additional benefits that supplementation can offer. No matter what supplementation you choose, you should follow these two guidelines:

- *Only buy from reliable sources:* Look for reputable third-party companies that are quality assured with classifications such as these: GMP Quality, USDA Organic, and Non-GMO Project Verified. For a detailed and complete listing on how to ensure pure and clean nutrition, go to my website at NaomiWhittel.com.

- *Only buy organic or wild-crafted plant and herbal supplements:* Because many herbal supplements are less likely to have third-party verification, buying organic helps to ensure that you're getting herbs that are free of pesticides. As someone who has experienced heavy-metal herbal poisoning, I urge you to ensure that all your herbal supplements are carefully tested for contaminants.

I recommend you consider a few essential nutrients, particularly since many of us already have greater deficiencies in them.

## VITAMIN D$_3$

Vitamin D$_3$ is a fat-soluble vitamin that acts like a hormone in the body, impacting all of our cells. Vitamin D$_3$ is very important for calcium metabolism since it helps us to absorb calcium in the digestive system, maintain calcium levels in the blood, and grow and maintain healthy bones. Having enough vitamin D$_3$ and calcium prevents rickets in children and osteomalacia in adults. Low levels of vitamin D$_3$ are also associated with osteoporosis.[1]

In the gut, vitamin D$_3$ is absorbed in the small intestine in the presence of fat. This is a win for the keto diet, because keto aids in the absorption of vitamin D$_3$ and other fat-soluble nutrients. It also assists in regulating cell growth by helping cells to grow when there is a wound to heal, stopping cells from growing in the case of cancer, and helping new cells to become a specific type of mature cell.[2] Vitamin D is vitally important for immune system function, supports insulin production, and helps with regulating blood pressure.

Here is the problem: as a country we are chronically and severely vitamin $D_3$ deficient.[3] The main reason is that we can't get all the vitamin $D_3$ we need from food. Although many High Fiber Keto foods such as salmon, mackerel, sardines, egg yolks, and grass-fed dairy products are at the top of the list for vitamin $D_3$ content, they do not make up for one part of the equation that many of us are missing: exposure to sunlight.

We have the ability to make vitamin $D_3$ in our skin, but we need enough of the right kind of sunlight to do it. The production is dependent on UVB radiation, so our geography plays a role. And our ability to synthesize, absorb, and metabolize vitamin $D_3$ may depend on skin pigmentation, genetics, age, and health status.

Many of us spend a lot of time indoors or live too far north to get adequate sun exposure for much of the year, and when we do go outside, we prevent vitamin $D_3$ from forming by covering up or wearing sunscreen to protect from skin cancer and other diseases. However, this has led to widespread vitamin $D_3$ deficiency. Supplementation can help to fill the gap between how much vitamin $D_3$ we need and how much we get. One of my favorite ways to supplement vitamin $D_3$ is with herring oil, such as Romega Arctic Caviar Oil, because along with the important omega-3 fats, herring oil is a natural source of both vitamin $D_3$ and choline.

**When and how much to take:**

- Most labs and physicians will consider blood levels of vitamin $D_3$ (25 hydroxy vitamin $D_3$) over 30 ng/mL to be sufficient, but evidence suggests that higher levels around 50 ng/mL are needed for optimal health.[4]

- It is important to work with your doctor to determine the level that is best for you as an individual and how much supplementation you need to get there.

# OMEGA-3S

Omega-3 fatty acids are a well-known category of polyunsaturated fats because of their anti-inflammatory properties.[5] Polyunsaturated refers to the chemical structure, as *poly* means many and *unsaturated* refers to double bonds.

Omega-3 fats play a key role in cell membranes and cellular communication, support cholesterol balance by increasing HDL ("good") cholesterol and reducing triglycerides, improve brain health and cognition, support healthy weight, and balance mood, all while reducing inflammation.

Here are three very important omega-3 fats to include in your diet:

*Alpha-linolenic Acid (ALA)* is considered the "essential" omega-3 fat because we cannot make it ourselves and it needs to be obtained from the diet.[6] The body can convert ALA into EPA and DHA, but this conversion level is quite low, and many experts agree that it is important to obtain EPA and DHA from the diet. ALA is found in flaxseeds, chia seeds, walnuts, hemp seeds, and algae.

*Eicosapentaenoic Acid (EPA)* is the omega-3 fat responsible for your body's anti-inflammatory properties.[7] Cells can turn EPA into a messenger (eicosanoid) molecule to signal surrounding cells to both shut off their inflammatory response and balance out their more inflammatory messages coming from omega-6 fats.

*Docosahexaenoic Acid (DHA)* is the omega-3 fat that is important for brain health and cognition.[8] It is essential for mothers to have enough DHA during pregnancy and nursing to provide their babies with these important fats for brain development.

EPA and DHA are found together in the same keto foods, and good sources include salmon, herring, sardines, mackerel, cod, scallops, oysters, and other seafood. Small amounts are also found in pasture-raised egg yolks, dairy, and beef.

Omega-3s may seem pretty straightforward, but as a whole, our omegas are out of balance. The standard American diet is way too high in omega-6 fats, primarily from processed vegetable oils, such as corn, soy, and safflower, and too low in omega-3 fats from whole nuts, seeds, and seafood. The recommended ratio of omega-6 to omega-3 fats is 4:1 or 2:1, depending on the subpopulation, and many Western diets are as high as 50:1 or even 200:1.[9]

While you need both omega-6 and omega-3 fats, it's clear that balance is key. On your High Fiber Keto plan, you'll naturally get enough omega-6 fats from high-quality whole foods such as poultry, meat, nuts, and seeds. Your 22-day program has been designed to optimize your omega-6 to omega-3 ratio by including salmon, other low-toxicity fatty fish, and mineral-rich seafood. All of which can work quickly to reduce inflammation in the body!

However, if you don't like fish or seafood, don't have access to high-quality sources, or have high levels of inflammation in your body, you will likely benefit from supplementing with additional omega-3 fats.

Omega-3 fats are quite fragile and can easily go rancid when exposed to light or heat, and it is very important to avoid ingesting rancid fats because they are inflammatory and cause damage to the body. Store omega-3 fats in a dark container in the fridge and discard when expired or if they smell rotten or rancid.

**When and how much to take:**

- 1 gram (1000 mg) per day of EPA plus DHA is a good general or maintenance dose.

- For therapeutic dosages for certain health concerns, 2 to 3 grams per day might be appropriate. Be sure to consult with your doctor or dietitian about the best dosage for you.

For anyone who has trouble digesting fats, taking digestive enzymes along with the supplements can be helpful. Omega-3 supplements are best tolerated with food.

# POWERPHENOLS

I have spent much of the last 10 years learning how to thrive *and* optimize my biology in a world where I often do 16-hour days. Being a mother of four and a CEO and founder of my own company, I need the best possible "go-tos" for myself and my family. I consider myself a bio-optimizer and have found what I believe to be the most powerful nutrients with the maximum benefits for our health and well-being.

I was led to these amazing nutrients after learning of the French paradox, the low occurrence of heart disease among the French, despite their consumption of high-fat foods. Red wine has been studied as a factor in that paradox. I then learned from the great minds about the protective power of polyphenols, such as those in red wine, that give plants their color and protect them from aggressors such as UV rays, insects, and disease. Among the 500-plus polyphenols that exist, there are four (trans-resveratrol, organic curcumin, berberine, and EGCG from green tea) that are incredibly potent. I termed them *Powerphenols.*

These four formidable plant extracts are proven to protect your cells and activate autophagy to repair them as well. They are powerfully effective at preventing cell oxidation and fighting cellular aging and reduce the risk of diabetes, cardiovascular disease, cancers, and neurodegenerative diseases. Furthermore, this unique combination of antioxidants has been shown to boost beneficial bacteria in your gut and optimize your metabolism so you have more energy while eating fewer calories.

Even though I've incorporated Powerphenols into the meal plan, because you'll be limiting many fruits and starchy vegetables, it is even more essential for you to maximize your intake of these four antioxidants. Here's why:

*Trans-resveratrol:* Every time you've ever enjoyed red wine, dark chocolate, or peanut butter, you're getting resveratrol, a Powerphenol found in grape skins and other plant sources, including peanuts, raspberries, and cocoa powder. Resveratrol, specifically trans-resveratrol, helps slow the aging process and helps to suppress many of the issues that contribute to metabolic dysfunction by enhancing mitochondrial function. It can also help reduce body weight and fat mass by controlling your appetite, lower blood glucose in patients with type 2 diabetes, reduce the proliferation of fat cells, decrease the production of stored fat, and reduce your risk of heart disease.[10]

*Organic curcumin:* This bright yellow phytonutrient derived from the turmeric plant wards off bacteria, fights depression, and may delay the effects of aging. It's a powerful anti-inflammatory and helps to regulate and improve insulin's ability to bind to sugar, reduces the activity of certain liver enzymes that release sugar into your bloodstream, and reduces total cholesterol, LDL ("bad") cholesterol, and triglycerides.

As mentioned, I always suggest that you buy organic when possible, but particularly for curcumin, since it's extracted directly from the turmeric root and you want to avoid getting any herbicides or pesticides that could have been absorbed by the plant through the roots.

*Berberine:* Extracted from certain plants, such as barberry and goldenseal, this Powerphenol is extremely difficult to find in food. I supplement daily with it and believe that berberine is a true superstar.

One of its many benefits includes activating AMPK (AMP-activated protein kinase), an enzyme often referred to as the "metabolic master switch"[11] because once activated, your cells neither make nor store fat. Instead, berberine spurs thermogenesis, a process by which brown adipose tissue uses fat in order to create heat to keep your body warm. The more often thermogenesis is triggered, the more calories you can burn by just standing still.

Berberine has also been shown to have a positive effect on your gut flora, which can help to ease digestive issues that arise when transitioning into a ketogenic diet. The compound is great for helping to fight off bacteria, viruses, and other harmful microorganisms and dramatically reducing blood sugar and cholesterol. Research[12] has shown that berberine's beneficial effects on blood sugar and lipid metabolism can be as effective as the prescription drug metformin and show great potential in treating type 2 diabetes, obesity, cardiac diseases, and inflammation.

*EGCG (epigallocatechin gallate):* This Powerphenol is found in high amounts in green tea and has been shown to suppress appetite, reduce fat, burn calories by helping to boost metabolism, and increase longevity by keeping your telomeres—the caps at the ends of your chromosomes—better protected against damage or fraying. From a metabolic perspective, the compound has been shown to break up the amyloid plaque in the brain that may be responsible for Alzheimer's disease and dissolve potentially dangerous protein plaques in your blood vessels, reducing your risk of heart attacks and stroke.[13]

**When and how much to take:**

- *Trans-resveratrol:* You can safely take up to 1,000 mg daily.

- *Organic curcumin:* Taking 500 mg twice a day is best, preferably with a fat-based meal to increase absorption.

- *Berberine:* I suggest taking three 500 mg doses a day with a meal.

- *EGCG:* It's safe for most adults to have up to 600 mg daily, spread out over three increments with meals to aid absorption.

Powerphenols are so important to helping provide the micronutrients that you are no longer getting in your diet due to the low levels of fruits and berries. However, you don't need to take all the Powerphenols together, and while I have suggested the dosages for the individual Powerphenols, I encourage you to use the sources and supplements that work best for you. You can go to the Resources section for recommendations.

## PREBIOTICS

Probiotics are live microorganisms that provide health benefits when consumed. They can be created in the fermentation process, such as the living bacteria in yogurt. Prebiotics are the largely indigestible parts of foods that pass through your small intestine and undergo fermentation by your microbiome when they reach the large intestine. This internal fermentation process feeds the already existing good or commensal bacteria and helps in maintaining a healthy gut microbiome.

Because most people eat fewer low-carb veggies and more high-fat foods, studies suggest that the decrease in overall fiber intake on a standard ketogenic diet can potentially lead to a reduction in certain types of beneficial bacteria in the gut, particularly *Bifidobacteria* and *Escherichia*.[14] My carefully designed meal plan includes an array of fiber-rich foods to avoid this common keto pitfall, but a little extra attention in this area would be a good nutritional insurance policy. Following are some of my favorite prebiotics:

*Chicory root:* This member of the dandelion family contains the soluble fiber inulin, a prebiotic resistant to digestion and absorption that nourishes gut bacteria[15] in a way that helps to reduce your risk of obesity, type 2 diabetes, heart disease, and certain inflammatory diseases.[16]

*Jerusalem artichoke:* Also known as the "Earth apple," this species of sunflower is a powerful prebiotic and is even denser in inulin than chicory root. It is high in potassium and thiamine and has been shown to maintain healthy blood glucose levels, support the immune system,[17] and possibly prevent metabolic diseases such as type 2 diabetes.[18]

*Acacia gum (aka gum arabic):* Naturally sourced from the sap of the acacia tree, this highly soluble fiber promotes healthy levels of the probiotic strains *Bifidobacteria* and *Lactobacilli* and is used therapeutically to support symptoms of irritable bowel syndrome (IBS) and relieve constipation. It may also play a part in decreasing body mass index (BMI), regulating your blood pressure,[19] and encouraging weight loss.[20]

*Psyllium:* Made from the seed husks of the *Plantago ovata* plant, this soluble fiber source is best known for its ability to work as a laxative. Psyllium has also been shown to lower fasting blood glucose and A1c levels in people with prediabetes and diabetes, as well as reduce LDL cholesterol.

*Green banana flour:* This natural flour alternative made from ground, unripe bananas is an incredible source of gut-friendly resistant starch, a special type of fermentable fiber that's been shown to decrease cholesterol and improve insulin sensitivity in those with metabolic syndrome.[21] Green bananas contain the amino acid 5-HTP, a key precursor to serotonin production that's been shown to increase feelings of satiety[22] and help treat depression,[23] insomnia, fibromyalgia, and migraines.[24]

*Glucomannan:* Derived from the root of the konjac plant, glucomannan (GM) is a supportive soluble fiber that can increase satiety and gut motility, which may help with weight loss. GM has also been found to reduce the glycemic load of foods and help to maintain healthy cholesterol levels.

*L-glutamine:* This amino acid helps fuel the cells within your small intestines to repair and recover, which is why it's so beneficial for reducing your risk of gastrointestinal (GI) inflammation and leaky gut. It supports the reduction of poor nutrient absorption and promotes proper fat digestion so that you're able to use more from every healthy nutrient you ingest.

**When and how much to take:**

- *Chicory root:* 2 tablespoons
- *Jerusalem artichoke:* 200 grams (about two small tubers) or about 2 grams of concentrated fiber
- *Acacia gum:* About 2 grams of concentrated fiber
- *Psyllium:* 5 grams (1 to 2 teaspoons of actual psyllium husk)
- *Green banana flour:* 2 tablespoons of flour or 2 grams of concentrated fiber
- *Glucomannan:* 2 grams
- *L-glutamine:* 2 grams

As I mentioned before, I encourage you to turn to whatever nutritional supplements you feel comfortable with. If you have Small Intestinal Bacterial Overgrowth (SIBO), certain gut infections, or dysbiosis, or know or suspect an infection or other underlying condition, always consult with your doctor before taking.

## ELECTROLYTES

I cannot overstate how important electrolytes are on a ketogenic diet. As you transition into nutritional ketosis, your body burns through stored glucose (glycogen). Because every gram of glycogen stores approximately 3 grams of water, your body also loses a lot of stored water, sodium, and other valuable electrolytes. In addition, once you switch to being a fat burner, your insulin levels naturally drop, which causes your kidneys to shed the stored sodium and water you've been holding on to from being a sugar burner.

If you're not careful to drink additional water or eat the green gel water veggies, the end result can be dehydration and an electrolyte imbalance, which can contribute to symptoms associated with keto flu. But far worse than that, not having enough of certain key electrolytes can play havoc with your metabolic health. That's because these mighty minerals are responsible for such functions as sustaining a healthy pH of fluids and tissues; moving nutrients into and toxins out of cells; and making certain that your nervous system, muscles, and brain all function properly. These are the five electrolytes that need to be equalized to ensure you maintain your metabolic edge:

> *Sodium:* Because much of the sodium in our diet today comes from consuming foods where salt is used as a preservative, it's a very misunderstood mineral. But as much as it's advised to restrict salt for health reasons, sodium is vital for helping your body's fluid maintenance, blood volume, and cellular pressure—keeping it all in balance

and functioning normally. Sodium also plays a role in protecting your body from depleting other electrolytes.

*Magnesium:* This important electrolyte has a hand in more than 600 chemical reactions that occur in your body, helps move other electrolytes in or out of your cells, and is a key mineral that helps muscles relax. Because my nutritional plan is abundant in dark leafy green vegetables that are a major source of magnesium, you will be getting a good amount. However, due to large-scale industrial agriculture practices, much of the soil has become depleted of magnesium, which may be why magnesium is one of the most common nutrient deficiencies in the world—and why I highly recommend supplementing it in a variety of forms.

*Potassium:* Although it is critical for maintaining healthy blood pressure, heart health, bone health, and muscle function, less than 3 percent of Americans ever hit the optimal daily amount for adults of about 4.7 grams. And because many high-potassium foods (such as bananas, potatoes, fruit juices, and beans) are eliminated on a ketogenic diet since they're also high carb, potassium becomes that much more important to pay special attention to.

*Calcium:* Even though you probably associate this mineral with your bones, a small amount also lives in your blood and is tightly regulated in order to help contract muscles, maintain the rhythm of your heart, and clot your blood. When following my plan, you'll meet your body's calcium needs through dairy and dark leafy greens. However, because of calcium's importance and synergy with sodium, magnesium, and potassium, adding it into your daily routine is a smart choice.

*Iodine:* Iodine is converted by your body into thyroid hormones, which are essential for controlling the speed of your metabolism.[25] In my meal plan, sea salt is the primary salt source because it contains small amounts of naturally occurring iodine and other trace minerals.

You'll also get this trace element from fish, seafood, egg yolks, yogurt, and seaweed.

**When and how much to take:**

Take each electrolyte at its recommended quantity three times per day. If you are on a salt-restricted diet for medical reasons, take medications for hypertension or cardiovascular disease that interact with sodium or potassium supplementation, are salt sensitive, or have a thyroid condition or kidney disease, consult with your doctor before taking supplements.

- *Sodium:* 100 to 700 mg (from sodium chloride or from sea salt or seawater, for a daily total of 300 to 2,100 mg)
- *Magnesium:* 100 mg (from magnesium citrate, for a daily total of 300 mg)
- *Potassium:* 300 mg (from potassium chloride, for a daily total of 900 mg)
- *Calcium:* 35 mg (from calcium chloride, for a daily total of 105 mg)
- *Iodine:* 70 mg (from potassium iodide or kelp, for a daily total of 210 mg)

## ENZYMES

Even though my meal plan naturally supports healthy digestion, having some additional enzymatic support when transitioning to a low-carb, high-fat diet can be extremely beneficial. Digestive enzymes—the substances that help break down food into smaller particles so that they can be digested and absorbed more easily by your body—are synthesized and secreted in such places as your mouth, stomach, pancreas, and intestines.

As you increase your fat intake, it's even more important to have the right type and amount of digestive enzymes. If you're not able to properly break down fats, becoming keto-adapted can become a much longer and more arduous process and can result in a variety of digestive issues, including gas, bloating, constipation, diarrhea, and nausea. When looking for a high-quality digestive enzyme, keep the following ingredients in mind for evaluating if the product is properly designed to optimize the breakdown of proteins, fats, carbs, and fiber, as well as determining whether it can effectively help you assimilate nutrients without indigestion, bloating, or cramps. There are many unique enzyme blends that can become your trusted sources for a comfortable transition into nutritional ketosis. I suggest looking for a broad-spectrum digestive enzyme that provides comprehensive support to all major phases of digestion. Here is my cheat sheet of the ingredients to look for:

*Fat-digesting enzymes:* Your body naturally produces *lipase*, the main fat-digesting enzyme, in your mouth, stomach, and pancreas to break down fat into glycerol and smaller fatty acids. Because the ketogenic diet is high in fat, digestive enzymes like *lipase* and *pepsin* are absolutely essential to have in ample amounts.

*Protein-digesting enzymes: Bromelain* is a mixture of protein-digesting enzymes. These enzymes, called *proteases*, support your body by breaking down proteins into their building blocks of amino acids, which are later absorbed through the small intestine.

*Dairy-digesting enzymes:* Because some of the high-fat foods you'll be enjoying are dairy based, having enough *lactase*—the enzyme responsible for digesting lactose, the naturally occurring sugar found in dairy—is key. Without *lactase*, you will likely become lactose intolerant, which will make enjoying most dairy products an unpleasant experience.

*Starch- and sugar-digesting enzymes: Amylase, beta-glucanase, cellulase, xylanase, glucoamylase, pectinase, hemicellulase,* and *invertase* are a group of enzymes essential for breaking down the plant cell walls from the abundance of fiber-rich foods you'll be eating on the program.

*Alpha-galactosidase:* This enzyme breaks apart sugar attached to a protein (glycoprotein) along with sugar attached to fat (glycolipid) and has been shown to reduce gas, bloating, and other symptoms that can arise from enjoying high-fiber foods.

*Phytase:* This unique enzyme breaks down phytic acid commonly found in certain plant foods, including non-keto options like legumes (lentils and beans) and whole grains (oats, quinoa, rice), and also popular keto foods like most nuts and seeds. Breaking down the phytic acid helps your body to absorb as much of the vitamins, minerals, and other nutrients as possible.

*Bacillus coagulans:* This beneficial probiotic bacteria works in conjunction with digestive enzymes to reduce your risk of excess gas, bloating, diarrhea, and constipation.

*Ginger:* Ginger aids in digestion, reduces gas, and has been used throughout history as an herbal remedy for nausea, which is a potential short-term side effect during the beginning phase of your transformation to becoming a fat burner. As your body becomes a fat-burning machine, it begins to build its team, and one integral member is a strong digestive presence. But as with all beginnings, sometimes we need a little help making the adjustment, and this is where ginger comes in really handy. Ginger assists the body in producing the bile that is necessary for the proper digestion and absorption of fat, decreases symptoms of reflux, and improves gut motility so that food can move through your GI tract with ease.

*Turmeric:* One of my all-time favorite spices for taste and overall health is turmeric. The bioactive component in this spice is *curcumin,* which plays a vital part in reducing inflammation of the digestive tract resulting from infections, irritable bowel syndrome, irritable bowel disease, and other inflammatory conditions that impact the mucus membrane of the GI tract. Turmeric also reduces gas and bloating and stimulates bile production in the liver, aiding fat digestion.

*Fennel:* Known for its distinct licorice taste, this plant supports digestive health; relaxes muscles of the digestive tract; and reduces gas, bloating, cramping, and constipation, which is why certain cultures chew fennel seeds or drink a fennel tea after meals. Fennel also stimulates stomach acid production and pancreatic enzymes.

*Apple cider vinegar (ACV), raw:* Used for centuries in cooking and cleaning and for medicinal purposes, this superfood stimulates enzyme and stomach acid production and acts as a powerful antimicrobial agent that kills pathogens and bacteria.[26] Studies have also shown that ACV may even support weight loss by raising AMPK,[27] lowering the storage of fat,[28] and reducing appetite.[29]

You absolutely do not have to take every single one of these supplements, but to start I recommend simply taking vitamin $D_3$ and omega-3s. But even taking no supplements at all, following the High Fiber Keto plan will give you plenty of benefits. For a list of recommended products, please see the Resources section.

To take these benefits a step further the next chapter will show you how simple movements can truly maximize your efforts when combined with the nutritional meal plan.

Note: If you know or suspect an intestinal blockage, have an allergy to any of the ingredients, or have or have had a stomach or intestinal tract ulcer, operation, or intestinal resection, consult with your health provider before taking supplements.

# ERIN

### *A game changer.*

I started keto when I was 33 after being on the typical low-fat, high carb diet for *way* too long. I found myself with anxiety, depression, fatigue, binge eating, never feeling satisfied, hormone imbalance (lost my period), and lack of sex drive. I had no idea it was related to the lack of fat until someone gave me a coffee with MCT oil and butter. It was almost like I turned into (poof!) Cinderella, and all my symptoms turned around.

Over the past year I noticed my gut needed some TLC. I was feeling sluggish and bloated, and it turns out I'm not the best at digesting fats! Going on the High Fiber Keto plan took me to the next level. It was amazing to me how incorporating a digestive enzyme, adding a prebiotic, more fiber from green veggies, and adding sea salt to everything, could make such a difference. I felt *so* much better. My gut issues and bloating were almost instantly gone. My tummy is flat . . . and that's a *first* time for me *ever*! Supplementing my keto diet has been a game changer and can really make all the difference when it comes to getting the results that you want!

# CHAPTER SEVEN

# MAKE YOUR METABOLISM MOVE

## The Fitness Plan to Get Your Energy System Going in the Right Direction

With all the roles you play and obligations you have, I know there is a lot on your plate (fiber included!). While some of you may have hit a nice groove with a regular exercise routine, others may feel like it's challenging to integrate *another* thing into your daily schedule.

Instead of lifting weights, maybe you're feeling the weight of responsibility. Instead of burning calories, maybe you're burning the candle at both ends. And instead of your regular sweat sessions, maybe your world is full of stress sessions.

Here's the great thing about the approach to exercise in my 22-day plan. It's simply about moving parts—yours!

Because adjusting to a new eating style can be difficult enough, I don't want you to worry about trying to integrate "formal" exercise in these first three weeks. Instead, I want to you to focus on an important metabolism-booster—just regular movement throughout the day.

Growing up in Europe, movement was always a big part of my life. Back then, I was so fortunate to be able to spend each of my summers living with my grandfather in the South of France. Not a single day went by when the two of us weren't walking around together visiting friends in a small village in the Provence region or just being up and about, doing some sort of chore or task.

I never considered how all that moving around might have been good for me, because as tired as I might have felt some days, it never felt like too much to handle, and it definitely never seemed like exercise. All I knew was that I was having fun, enjoying nature, and being active from sunup to sunset.

My grandfather was (and still is) a smart man, so he might have always been wise to the power of movement. In fact, I'm pretty sure he was. Because at 93 years young, he's still as healthy and energetic as ever and continues to work on research as a physicist with a mind as sharp as it was when I was young. And here's the surprising part: he's never officially set foot in a gym. That's because even though I'm no longer around to tag along with him as I once did, to this day, he still *moves* as often as possible from sunup to sunset.

But as much as I loved all that moving, eventually life just got in the way. I'll always remember those days fondly, but according to science, nothing misses all that moving around more than metabolism.

Consider these two important facts:

*Movement has become M.I.A.* It may seem that we're always on the move, but the truth is that we're not really moving as much as we should. We get so swallowed up by the obligations we have to our families, jobs, and everything else around us that we often have less opportunity to be active, or we feel guilty about focusing on ourselves. Even when we *do* allow ourselves those precious "me moments," it's hard not to want to just unwind and relax instead of using that time wisely by getting up and moving more. But according to leading physical-activity and healthy-aging expert Heather Hausenblas, Ph.D., perhaps the mistake we have made is how we've engineered regular movement out of our lives through innovation and technology—and how we think that intense exercise is the only and best solution.

According to Dr. Hausenblas, we've made things so easy for ourselves that we're losing time once spent on "incidental physical activity." When you take these tiniest of movements away—say, using an electric toothbrush or can opener instead of doing these tasks manually—you begin to take away all these little moments of physical activity that add up over the course of weeks, months, and years. It's probably not too much of a stretch to say that the lack of activity coincides in part with the prevalence in obesity. Since 1980, it has doubled in more than 70 countries and has continued to increase in most other countries.[1]

So what we're going to do on the 22-day High Fiber Keto plan is get you to effortlessly sneak in the right amount of daily activity to develop an optimized metabolism without having to sacrifice much time at all.

*You can boost your metabolism without intense exercise.* I can't tell you how many women I've spoken to who have told me how they've become conditioned to look for that *typical* workout plan when starting any new lifestyle program. But when it comes to getting your metabolism on track, the answer isn't always found through hours in a weight room. It's what you're doing when you're just waiting around that offers the biggest bang for your metabolic buck.

Your body primarily burns calories in three ways. First, it burns them just to keep you alive and functioning. Second, it burns them to digest the foods you eat, which is referred to as the *thermic effect of food*.[2] (Yes, that's right—you actually burn calories as you eat calories!) And third, it burns them to fuel activity, otherwise known as *activity thermogenesis*.[3]

This last one—these are the calories you burn whenever you exercise—and what so many women desperately count on when they want to lose weight, improve their cardiovascular strength, or reverse metabolic syndrome. Although the science is very clear that you need to get your heart rate up a little bit each day at a moderate to vigorous level,[4] there are many women out there whom Hausenblas refers to as "active couch potatoes." These are women who meet the physical activity guidelines by getting about 30 minutes of exercise daily, yet spend the rest of their day in sedentary activities like sitting. They can still experience myriad health issues.

I understand why the right type and amount of movement has become a missing piece of the metabolic puzzle for most women—and I have been equally guilty of losing that piece. But I have discovered it's possible to sneak in the right amount of daily activity needed to enjoy an optimized metabolism without investing money or time in equipment, memberships, or classes. You can regain an optimized metabolism through movement, and it's all about transforming your mind-set about the definition of movement.

That's because activity thermogenesis is a two-way street. Yes, your body burns calories when you exercise. But you actually burn an overwhelming number of your total daily calories when you're not exercising at all in non-exercise activity thermogenesis, or NEAT.[5]

According to Dr. Hausenblas, whenever you're working, walking, dancing, shopping, and just standing around doing absolutely nothing, you're burning calories and improving your metabolic health—and that's NEAT. In fact, the number of calories NEAT burns can range from about 15 percent to as much as 50 percent or more of your daily energy expenditure, even if you don't presently exercise.[6] When you focus on movement all day long—and not just that moment in the gym or during a workout—you're removing as many instances of inactivity from your day as possible.

Let me ask you something, which person would you rather be? The one that has to drive to the gym to spend an hour sweating through their shirt, pressing a weight off their chest with a movement that we don't do anywhere else—or the one who goes about their normal day, eating, relaxing, and moving only to do what needs to be done?

You see, optimizing your metabolism can mean tweaking how you *already* move, stand, and sit throughout your day. You can take advantage of NEAT to burn even more calories and increase your opportunity to optimize metabolism.[7]

And as we prepare to launch into the 22-day plan, you will see exactly how you can use it to optimize your metabolism.

## THE "ME-TIME" THAT MAGNIFIES METABOLISM

For the next 22 days, you'll follow the same "metabolic movement" makeover that participants in my clinical trial used to ignite the power of NEAT all day long to give them an optimized metabolism. I call it *ME-Time*, short for *Metabolic-Edge Time*. It's a simple, three-part approach that increases your physical activity, decreases your sedentary behavior, and turns moments of inactivity (when you have little choice but to stand or sit) into what Dr. Hausenblas refers to as *active sedentary behavior* or *low-active behavior*,[8] meaning you will burn extra calories and raise your metabolism during moments when your metabolism typically drops due to inactivity.

Each day along your High Fiber Keto journey will include these actions:

- *You will* step *up* . . . by walking a minimum of 7,500 steps per day

- *You will* stand *up* . . . by never sitting longer than 30 minutes at any given time

- *You will* shake *up* . . . by engaging in some form of active sedentary behavior as often as possible (such as tapping your feet or fingers, shaking your hands or legs, moving around in your chair, or any type of movements done while either standing or seated)

Super simple, right? It is, and that's just one reason I love ME-Time. Not only is it effective at combating metabolic syndrome, but because of ME-Time's simplicity, it's within everyone's reach. And when something isn't a huge stretch, it's much easier to incorporate into the regular routine in your life.

That's exactly what I want for you. My hope is that after 22 days, you'll no longer be consciously aware of the need to move more—you'll simply move more without even realizing it by turning these tactics into tried-and-true habits. My greatest wish is that these changes eventually become so much a part of who you are that you never have to return to this chapter to remember what you have to do—because you'll be doing it subconsciously, all day long, for the rest of your life. And I also hope that you will rethink movement in a way that will make it impossible *not* to turn every motion into an optimized metabolism.

However, simplicity isn't the only reason this minimalistic metabolism-boosting approach is so effective.

> **It's custom fit for nutritional ketosis.** Can you imagine figuring out your taxes while running on a treadmill? Can you picture writing a report for your boss while skipping rope? My point: It pays to step away from traditional exercise (just for a little while) until you've got everything figured out. Because if you don't, the mistakes you might make by overwhelming yourself are never worth it.

The same principle applies to nutritional ketosis. As you switch over from using glucose to the much cleaner fuel of ketones and fat, everything within your body will begin to adapt and transform at the same time—and at a very rapid pace.[9] From your hydration levels and mineral concentrations to the ratio of good versus bad bacteria within your microbiome, a metabolic systematic change will occur. And if you add exercise that's too intense to the equation, it could have a negative effect on your body's ability to adjust to this optimized metabolism. That's why integrating this simple yet efficient movement approach is the smarter choice during the 22-day plan.

> **It's cost effective.** You only need supportive footwear and a quality pedometer (which can be provided by an app on your smartphone or costs between $3 and $20 for a separate device). There's no need for a gym membership, new clothes, exercise equipment, or any additional investment whatsoever.

> **It's subconscious exercise.** It's exercise on autopilot, where the act of moving more will simply be what you

do all day long without ever giving it a second thought or breaking a sweat!

**It's recovery friendly.** Dr. Hausenblas stresses that when it comes to incorporating movement into your life each and every day, you should never feel the need to recover, meaning you should never feel so tired or sore afterward that you couldn't perform the same exact movements the very next day if asked to. ME-Time does not ask you to engage in intense or extreme amounts of activity that will require your body to take time off in order to recover. That's what makes ME-Time so efficient. Even though you'll be raising your metabolism through movement, you'll never be pushing yourself to a point where you won't be able to ask your body to do it again tomorrow.

**It all adds up.** Getting in at least 150 minutes of movement a week benefits your health and significantly lowers your risk of developing metabolic syndrome.[10] The problem: Most of us try to hit that number by breaking it up into larger chunks, such as exercising for 30 minutes five times a week. However, if we miss or skip a session, it can cause a feeling of disappointment or need to make up that lost time.

The scientific truth is it doesn't matter whether you do all 150 minutes in a single session or spread those 150 minutes out by moving around for a few minutes at a time. It's the weekly volume (how many minutes you're active), not the frequency (how often you're active) that matters to your metabolism.[11] The beauty of ME-Time is that you'll accumulate that minimum number of 150 minutes in smaller doses throughout the week without stressing out throughout the day.

**It lets you move at your own pace.** The movements that make up ME-Time (walking, standing, and movement during sedentary activity) are movements that many people can do already—it's just that we don't do them as often as we should. That means there's zero learning curve. And if you have health challenges that limit your mobility, that's okay; you'll be able to start where *you* are and then build from there.

**It's instantly exhilarating.** According to Dr. Hausenblas, whenever you move around, there's an immediate improvement to both your mood and well-being. In fact, movement may be just as powerful as mindful meditation for lowering stress and anxiety.[12] So by moving all day long instead of working out and then being sedentary for the rest of the day, you'll increase the number of times per day where you feel better mentally and emotionally.

## STEP UP!

For 22 days, I want you to try to walk a minimum of 7,500 steps each day.

According to research, hitting a high daily step count on a regular basis lowers blood pressure,[13] lowers triglycerides,[14] and can lower your risk of all-cause mortality.[15] Furthermore, walking has been shown to improve many risk factors related to metabolic syndrome, including inflammation, cholesterol, mental stress, obesity, and vascular stiffness.[16]

But let's face it, getting in 7,500 steps every single day isn't always easy. However, this sweet spot for steps is less of an effort than it may seem since we will be focusing more on *how* you spend your time moving and less about the mileage.

According to researchers out of Oregon State University, even if you can't hit 10,000 steps, walking fewer steps but moving at a higher cadence (100 steps per minute) is still beneficial to your well-being.[17] In addition, approximately 7,000 to 8,000 steps per day meets the minimum amount of moderate-to-vigorous activity (MVPA) required by current public health activity guidelines to achieve optimal health benefits.[18]

**What if you can't do 7,500 steps?** That's entirely fine. If you are able, I'd love to see you hit that 7,500-step goal every day. But that's not possible for everyone.

The magic of my movement program is that you have the freedom to start at the right level for your body—whether it's with steps or other types of movement. In the next chapter, I'll show you how to discover how many "baseline steps" you typically walk each day, as well as how to test what you're capable of with "boost steps." After that, you'll know the average number of steps per day that's best for *you*—and that's where you will start. Then you can keep building from there.

Once you have a sense of how many steps you can do, you'll build on that number every few days throughout the 22-day program in a way that's both comfortable and wise for your body.

If at any time you find yourself feeling overly tired or sore after increasing your step count, then I want you to lower your steps back down to where they were before and stay there for a few more days to give your body more time to acclimate before raising your count again.

For example, if you were walking 5,000 steps each day, then raised it to 5,300 steps and felt overly exhausted or sore the next day, go back to doing 5,000 steps for a few more days and see how you feel.

Finally, if you never build up to 7,500 steps by the end of the program, I want you to do two things for me. One, feel proud of yourself because you're technically at a better metabolic place than when you began. It's really that simple.

And two, I want you to remember that ME-Time is a rethinking of movement that I want you to absorb for life. So even if you never quite reached 7,500 steps, you have a lifetime to accomplish that goal. Even if it's one step at a time, the more you build up that number, the more you'll gain an optimized metabolism. Best yet, the longer you stay in an optimized state, the easier it will become for you to reach that 7,500-step goal.

**What if 7,500 is too easy?** Instead of adding more steps, what I want you to do is speed up the cadence to a pace of 100 steps per minute (you can equate 100 steps per minute to walking a 20-minute mile) for at least 30 minutes each day.[19] These 30 minutes of faster steps don't have to be all at once and can easily be broken up throughout your day. By performing a certain number of steps at a higher cadence, you'll not only finish in less time, but you'll boost the intensity and make those steps more metabolically effective.

Tip: Use a pedometer app on your smartphone to calculate your walking cadence.

But what should you do if you already walk that fast? First, know that's amazing because that means you're already moving at a moderate pace. Raising the intensity by walking even faster can get tricky because vigorous walking is a pace of 130 steps per minute, and jogging starts at 140 steps per minute.

For now—and only if you feel fit enough and don't experience any soreness or fatigue that prevents you from walking each and every day—you can experiment with walking at a cadence of between 110 to 120 steps per minute for at least 30 minutes each day. Or you can maintain your pace of 100 steps per minute and reach for 10,000 steps per day.

**What if you want to do even more?** Dr. Hausenblas confirms that the more steps you do, the better it can be for you—but up to a point. The research is clear that people who engage in regular physical activity between 150 and 300 minutes per week significantly reduce their risk of just about every chronic disease conceivable, from cancer and obesity to diabetes and cardiovascular disease.[20]

But once you go over 300 minutes per week, Dr. Hausenblas says that even though there can be performance benefits if you're an athlete, the additional health benefits from activity are very minimal. After 300 minutes, there's a diminished return because you run the risk of actually exercising too much,[21] which can lead to overtraining and cause constant muscle soreness, elevated levels of cortisol, stress, trouble sleeping, joint pain, digestion issues, moodiness, and anxiety.[22]

All of that being said, every body is different. So if you feel the need to go beyond 10,000 steps, make sure to ask yourself the following questions:

- Is my body trying to tell me *no*? (Listen for the signs of overtraining—such as chronic muscle soreness, achy joints, feeling run down, or difficulty sleeping—and if you experience any, then know that it's time to pull back.)

- Am I being unrealistic? (Sometimes, we may want to do more, even though we may not be physically or mentally ready. If that's you, just be patient and remember that exercising for an optimized metabolism is a lifelong journey—not a sprint.)

Ask yourself these questions each and every day. If you can honestly say *no* to both, then you can walk farther than 7,500 steps if you feel up to it. But if the answer is *yes* to either or both, then bring yourself back down to a step count that's safer and more manageable for the time being.

### How to Step Up More Often

Achieving your daily step goal doesn't have to be monotonous, and you don't have to walk around for the sake of walking. Of course, take a stroll and enjoy your surroundings if you want, especially if you can get someone to join you. But reaching that tally doesn't have to be something you have to plan or carve out time for. Instead, it can easily be achieved simply by going about your day—in a slightly smarter way.

There are many tricks you can use to add more steps without having them steal time away from what you need to do. As a matter of fact, when done right, it's possible to hit that number *and* accomplish a lot more for yourself by getting tasks done, bonding with family and friends, and basically staying ahead of your life. It becomes a matter of not counting steps, but making every step count.

**Look for the long cuts.** What's a long cut, you ask? Easy—it's the opposite of a shortcut! It's only natural to always seek out the shortest path or fewest number of trips whenever we run an errand, perform a task, or go about our day. Instead, try adding a few steps to every task or breaking things up a in a way that leaves you little choice but to step things up.

- Instead of bringing in several shopping bags from the car in one trip, bring in one bag at a time.

- Pick the farthest (but still safe) parking spot you can from where you need to visit.

- Instead of always walking straight toward where you need to go, circle around to it.

- Make a point to walk up to someone to talk instead of calling out to them—that isn't polite anyway!

**Whenever you talk—always walk.** Whether it means pacing back and forth when you're on the phone or inviting someone to take a walk with you if they want to speak with you, try making a hard-and-fast rule that if your lips are moving, then your feet must follow.

**Take it outside.** Dr. Hausenblas agrees with me that when people move outside into green space (trees and grass), their mood improves. And when you couple that with "blue space" (any body of water), their mood improves even more.[23] A recent report drawn from more than 140 studies involving 290 million people worldwide has conclusively shown that being exposed to green space more often reduces your risk of type 2 diabetes, cardiovascular disease, stress, and high blood pressure.[24]

**Forgive yourself.** Nobody is perfect, and life has a way of upsetting even the best-laid plans. If for some reason or another, you find that hitting your step goal on a certain day is impossible, just dust yourself off and try your best tomorrow. Feeling guilty is not the goal of this program, and I promise, those fewer steps today won't derail you from achieving an optimized metabolism tomorrow.

## STAND UP!

For 22 days, I also want you to concentrate on standing more. And by that, I mean stand as often as possible—all day long. But in the event that you do find yourself having to sit for any extended period of time because of your job, social engagements, watching TV, or being up in the bleachers cheering on your kids, that's fine. In these moments, I want you to stand up and move around for a minimum of 1 to 2 minutes every 30 minutes. During that time, I encourage you to do whatever you wish—walk around, hop in place, do standing squats or lunges, or just stand still—but I want you up and out of your seat.

The very first time I had the pleasure to interview Dr. Hausenblas for my docuseries *The Real Skinny on Fat*, we discussed how sitting is now regarded by many in the medical field as the new smoking because of its negative effects on our overall health and well-being. Large-scale meta-analyses have shown that people who sit more during the day are at a greater risk of most chronic diseases. Spending too much time sitting has been linked to high blood pressure, high cholesterol, heart disease, an increased waist circumference, and obesity, in addition to other health concerns, including type 2 diabetes, cancer, osteoporosis, and depression.

But the running list of why sitting is so serious doesn't stop there. Recent research has revealed that excess sitting may increase the risk of conditions you may never have considered before, such as accelerated aging. Research out of the University of California, San Diego, School of Medicine found that elderly women who sit more than 10 hours a day have cells that are eight years biologically older than their actual chronological age.[25] All that time spent on your bottom may even affect your brain, and UCLA researchers are currently looking into how constant sitting may thin out certain regions of the mind, particularly related to memory formation.[26]

Yet, despite all that we know about the dangers of excess sitting, it doesn't seem to stop most of us from doing it. As of 2019, the average adult in America spends about six and a half hours a day sitting (up from five and a half hours since 2007), according to a recent analysis published in the *Journal of the American Medical Association*.[27] And it's believed that one in four adults go beyond that number, sitting for more than eight hours a day.

The good news is that all of these health risks can be reversed by standing up as often as you can. Dr. Hausenblas states that one of the many processes impacted by chronic sitting is metabolism, where sitting for longer than an hour causes your metabolism to significantly slow down. But the simple act of standing up—even for a couple of minutes—reinvigorates your metabolism just as quickly and burns calories at a rate of 0.15 calories per minute more than sitting.[28] That subtle difference can really add up. According to Dr. Hausenblas, some people have shed upward of 10 pounds during one year from doing nothing but standing more.

## How to Stand Up More Often

In order to make sure the participants in my trial stood more during the day, I followed a method similar to research that proved the effectiveness of using prompts to break up sedentary time for office workers.[29]

In my clinical study, participants were prompted to stand and move more through texts and e-mails sent between 9 A.M. and 6 P.M. every day. Every 30 minutes, they would receive a message on their screens that read, "Time to GET UP! If you're sitting, stand and walk for a minute. If you're unable to walk around, then stand. If you're unable to stand, try to move your body around as much as possible. You can do it!"

Some participants found that their own schedule of when to move and get up worked better for them, but ultimately, everyone was encouraged to find a way to increase their own movement each day. Participants were also sent a daily wellness survey every morning where they could self-report whether they felt they moved more or not. It allowed each participant to reflect on the day and individualize their increases from day to day.

Now, even though I can't be there for you in the same way, that doesn't mean you can't remind yourself to do the same. Using your smartphone alarm and setting it for 30 minutes—or downloading a time-management app that does the same—is the obvious solution. But there may be times when having an alarm going off is easier said than done. In those instances, there are a few ways to make it more convenient, or even automatic, to go from seated to standing without needing a friendly nudge.

### When at your desk

- Always stand when reading your emails—then sit when answering them.
- Stand whenever you find yourself looking to see what time it is.

### When watching TV

- Get up at every commercial break.
- Place the remote away from yourself so that you have to get up every time you want to change the channel or adjust the volume.

### When out socializing (at the movies, a game, or any type of event)

- Always choose the seat closest to the aisle so you can stand up and stretch without being bothersome.
- Be the one to offer to go to the snack bar.

### When on your smartphone

- Make a hard-and-fast rule to never sit when texting or checking your three favorite apps.

## SHAKE UP!

Last but not least, for 22 days I want you to engage in some form of active sedentary behavior whenever you have little to no choice but to stay, sit, or stand in one place.

As much as I would love to have you walking about and always standing instead of sitting, I also know that for many of us, those two options are not always easy to pull off whenever we wish. Whether it's having to wait in line, sit in a meeting, or ride shotgun on a family road trip, there will be countless times when you'll simply be stuck in one spot.

But just because you can't move around doesn't mean you can't move around. There are many sedentary moments in our day that we don't typically think of as opportunities to have an effect on our metabolic health. Dr. Hausenblas has helped me understand how simple motions that you can do when you're sedentary—such as shaking your leg, tapping your fingers, or shifting in your seat—may not elevate your heart rate or work up a sweat but can still incrementally grant you an optimized metabolism. And the latest research shows us that small movements of the hands and feet while sedentary (what some call fidgeting or spontaneous movement) improve your health.[30]

Researchers at the University of Missouri theorize that fidgeting while sitting may potentially help prevent sitting-induced leg endothelial (blood vessel) dysfunction.[31] When subjects were asked to tap one foot for 60 seconds at a pace of 250 times per minute—but keep their other leg perfectly still—they discovered that the fidgeting leg had a significant increase in blood flow.

That's why for the purposes of my study, I asked the women that participated to engage in fidgeting behavior as often as possible during any periods of sedentary behavior throughout the day.

### How to Shake Up More Often

I get it. I really do. There's sometimes a stigma attached to appearing nervous, restless, or impatient because of never seeming to be able to sit or stand still. But there are many inconspicuous or socially acceptable ways to shake things up without necessarily catching people's eyes.

## While standing

- Shift your weight from one foot to the other, or sway from side to side.
- Take small steps forward and backward.
- Raise one foot slightly off the ground and hold it there for a few seconds, then switch to the other foot, continuing to alternate back and forth.
- Bend your knees a few inches and squat down. You can repeat this motion or squat down and hold the position for as long as you comfortably can. If you rub your thighs at the same time, you'll look like you're just stretching your legs.

## While sitting

- Rock back and forth or side to side, or rotate your torso in circles.
- With your toes planted on the floor, shake your legs up and down.
- If there's room, swing your legs back and forth, or bend and straighten them repeatedly.
- Drum your hands against the sides of your thighs.
- Think of a song and just allow yourself to move or dance in your seat.
- Try sitting on an exercise ball or something else that safely challenges your stability.

My goal is to (1) help you become more aware of consistent movement throughout the day and (2) put regular movement into action. The small steps when it comes to exercise will be a big part of how you get your metabolism working for you, and I hope this approach is easy to integrate into your life. My ultimate hope is that *your* moving parts will help you tackle *life's* moving parts with better health and more energy.

# NANCY

### *You + Keto = Success.*

Now that I am in my 40s, I get it. I get why women are confused about stubborn weight—why they accept the additional pounds every few years. I get why they're confused about what's happening with their skin. I get why they're tired and withdraw from activities they used to love. I get why we make the same conclusion: This is just what happens when we get older.

I never struggled with weight or skin or moods or fatigue—until I hit 37. Then my weight started creeping up. I was tired. Once an active person, I slowed my exercise down to the bare minimum. Even skin issues I never had before like eczema popped up.

And you know what my doctor told me? "Get over it" and that it was a normal part of aging.

I said to myself, *I don't think so.*

So I tried all kinds of things—cleanses, dieting using acupressure, counting macronutrients for heavy weight training, and restricted eating for "allergies."

Enter the next thing on my list . . . keto—to me, keto made sense. But my first foray into it was confusing, and I failed because I didn't understand the how, what, and when of eating.

But I couldn't get out of my head all the success stories I had read and the science behind it.

High Fiber Keto was easy to understand and manageable, and now I'm 14 pounds down and feel like I am back to myself. I have ramped up to exercising five days a week because I *want to.* Plus, I haven't seen the eczema creep back onto my hands since. This program helps you to ease into all the facets that makes You + Keto = Success. I'm happy. I don't even think about "cheating" and this is a way of life for me.

# CHAPTER EIGHT

# THE PRE-FIX PREP PLAN

## The Key to Success Lies in Execution *and* Preparation

Imagine that you are standing on the edge of your favorite body of water—a chilly yet enticing body of water. You have three choices:

- Say, "Heck no, I'm outta here."
- Dip your toes in, then your feet, then your legs, then your waist, until you slowly get accustomed to the water and put your full body in.
- Just jump on in.

This is exactly your choice with High Fiber Keto. I'll assume that choice 1 is not your choice since you're here and ready to take the plunge. But that still leaves a decision between choice 2 and choice 3.

While I might advise choice 3 when it comes to your favorite pool, lake, or ocean, that's not the best way to start a new diet or lifestyle. Jumping right in will set you up to have your breath taken away because it will be such a shock to your system. This, I would argue, is why so many diets fail. While your mind *wants* to jump in, the reality is that changing a way of eating takes more than just motivation; it takes some preparation. That's logistical prep, psychological prep, and nutritional prep.

So when it comes to preparing for my High Fiber Keto plan, it's a toes-knees-waist kind of approach, where you test the waters before you fully immerse yourself.

Success happens when you're well prepared.

Throughout my personal journey of trying to bridge the worlds of science and age-old wisdom with regard to health and well-being, I've truly felt grateful to learn from so many leading experts over the years. But the greatest lesson that keeps revealing itself along my path has been this:

*Those who make the greatest changes in life*
*never leap into change spontaneously.*

Asking you to switch from being a sugar burner to a fat burner without preparing you beforehand would be like making you take a test without studying—and expecting you to get an A.

I want the process of improving your metabolic health to work for you, and there are a few crucial steps that experts and the participants within my study revealed to me. These steps will help minimize and potentially eliminate the common problems and issues most people experience when switching to keto, consuming more fiber, and adding more movement into their day.

Before you begin the 22-day High Fiber Keto plan, I want you to give yourself at least two weeks to use these strategies so that you're primed in a way that lets you take advantage of the metabolic benefits available to you right from the start.

Ready to begin? Let's go!

## YOUR PRE-FIX KETO PLAN

Many people assume—and I'll admit, I was one of them—that before starting any ketogenic diet, it might make sense to modify what and how you eat to give your body a leg up on what to expect. After all, you're about to completely switch fuel sources—surely there's *something* you could eat or cut back on a week earlier to make that change less dramatic. Maybe you've considered preparing for the removal of carbs by gorging on them beforehand so you will miss them less. Or perhaps you've thought about how you could cut back on carbs a little at a time so it's not as much of a shock to your system when you heavily restrict them.

Neither is a good approach.

When it comes to switching fuel sources, you can eat whatever you wish right up until you start. In fact, in the professional opinion of ketogenic specialists Dr. Volk and Dr. Saenz, among others, it's advised *not* to make any major changes to your diet prior to the day you begin.

According to Dr. Volk, who personally handles medically supervised, highly strategic ketogenic approaches, if you begin this program after a day or more of carb bingeing, it shouldn't affect your ability to be successful in switching fuel sources. In addition, cutting back on carbs little by little before you start isn't doing your body the favor you think it is. As Dr. Volk explains, when you gradually reduce carbohydrates a little bit at a time, you may likely still experience the ups and downs that come with elevated blood sugar and insulin surges. You're also more susceptible to cravings, mood swings, and energy dips because your body is still running on carbs—but now you're giving your body even less to work with.

So when it comes to eating, it's best that you stay the course until you start Day 1. The notable exception is that you should integrate more fiber into your diet if you're typically low in fiber intake. In the meantime, there are a few things you can do prior to starting the plan that can make the transition as seamless as possible.

### Be smart—about when to start

Yes, you may be eager to begin the process as quickly as possible, and I really admire that enthusiasm and dedication. However, Dr. Volk has watched many people jump on board a ketogenic diet without giving their bodies enough time to adapt to switching fuel sources, only to end up hopping off because of other obligations.

I certainly understand how life can get in the way. That's why I want you to think ahead before you start my program. Is a major event in your life forthcoming? Are you in the midst of a situation making life more stressful than usual? If so, consider starting the program at another time, when everything feels relatively normal. But if you've decided that the time to begin is now, follow the rest of these tips to make sure you get to the starting line with the highest chance of success.

### Be prepared—to move forward

One of the best ways to prepare for a ketogenic diet is to organize your kitchen ahead of time.

- *Add what works for you:* In my plan, you'll find every meal *and* every ingredient you'll be eating for the next 22 days. So before you start, make sure that you have everything you need, especially for that first week. Understandably, you may not want to purchase certain cuts of meats or fish too soon since fresher is always better. But if shopping is not convenient for you, it's entirely fine to stock up on certain items and freeze them.

- *Remove what works against you:* Go through your pantry, refrigerator, and any place where you may have high-carb foods stored and find them another home. It is paramount to do a quick sweep for sugar and get rid of any temptations.

- *Resuscitate your spice rack:* Even if you find all the spices and herbs you'll need for the recipes in your cabinets, consider tossing the ones that may have outlived their usability. If kept in a cool, dark, and dry place, ground spices are usually good for about six months. After that, they may still smell nice but they're less potent. Take a look at your spices and herbs to make sure they are fresh and up to date.

## Be supported—by others

Do I believe that you have the strength to do this program without needing to rely on anyone else but yourself? Of course I do. But does the program become a much easier process when you have others who are supportive of you every step of the way? Without question. In fact, the support you surround yourself with before you begin and that you have along the way can sometimes mean the difference between staying the course and straying off the path.

Without the support of somebody reminding them how they're doing great or how eating a low-carb diet is what they should be doing, some people can lose motivation.[1] It can be helpful to have someone point out the positive, since it can be difficult to monitor your own progress.

That's why before you begin my program, I want you to let everyone around you—at home or at work, your friends, and anyone at any place you frequent often—know what you're about to embark on. Doing so makes you accountable. But more importantly, it helps you gauge others' potential for support before you begin. Sometimes the people we believe will support our efforts don't, while other times people we would have never expected to be supportive become our rocks. As you cast out your intentions to those around you, it will become instantly clear who to turn to if you need words of encouragement or advice.

## Be wiser—with your water

When your body runs on sugar, it stores carbohydrates in your liver and muscles in the form of glycogen.[2] Every gram of glycogen has about 3 or 4 grams of water attached to it. During the first initial stages of fat adaptation when your body is turning to stored glycogen for energy, you are releasing water at a higher rate. Electrolyte balance becomes affected and a common response is to lose water and electrolytes during the first days of carbohydrate restriction.

Even though my program is well formulated to make sure that you don't experience electrolyte losses, it's still critical that you stay hydrated. As Dr. Volk points out, a large portion of us tend to be chronically dehydrated in the first place.[3]

When I spoke to experts about how much water to drink each day, the answers varied because a person's individual needs also vary. But what was clear is that the typical "eight 8-ounce glasses of water" approach that's often recommended for the general public is too low when you're on keto. Instead, what many experts, including the Institute of Medicine, recommend is consuming between 91 and 125 ounces of water daily,[4] or approximately 11 to 15 glasses of water per day.

### Be ready—to argue with your brain

As you adjust to nutritional ketosis, you'll feel the satiety that comes from fat, meaning you will be full for longer and cravings may reduce.[5] Nonetheless, your brain can sometimes get in your way early in that process.

Being afraid of consuming fat and being told to eat every few hours has become so ingrained in our culture that it can be difficult to wrap your mind around eating higher amounts of fat and how satiated you'll be by consuming lower volumes of food in general. Even as you begin to feel better eating a different concentration of fat and calories, you may not be able to stop your brain from reminding you how contradictory it is to what you've always been told you would be feeling—and so you might quit. This is where having that support of someone is so crucial—someone who can talk with you, help you, and inspire you during times when you're uncomfortable.

### Be patient—and trust the process

Our bodies are highly complex systems, unique to every individual, so it may take anywhere from a few days to several weeks to even months for some people until your body becomes fully fat adapted. It isn't realistic to expect that you are going to feel incredible starting on Day 1.

Yet within the first weeks of doing keto, you may experience a dip in energy as your body acclimates. At this point you may think, *Something's not right here. I'm supposed to be feeling the benefits of nutritional ketosis, but it doesn't feel like I am—so I quit.*

If this is you, I want you to be patient and look at the situation in the same way you look at jet lag for a fun vacation. You may feel a little sluggish, and it may take a while to adjust, but it is *always* worth it.

## YOUR PRE-FIX MOVEMENT PLAN

Just as you need to prepare your body for nutritional ketosis, you need to get your body ready to move. But before you can do that, it helps to know how much you're moving already.

### Count—but don't critique or compete

Over 22 days, your goal will be 7,500 steps a day. That might be too many or too few steps for you right now. This is where we're going to find that out together.

**Baseline steps:** For three consecutive days, I want you to do a "baseline voyage" and get a clear sense of what an average day looks like for you when it comes to movement. Track your steps, but don't try to step more than usual. Allow yourself to remain oblivious to how many steps you're walking each day.

- *Make them normal days:* Your three baseline days should be three consecutive days that you consider to be routine. I don't want you to measure your baseline while on vacation, over the holidays, or during any type of special days where you might walk more or less than usual.

- *Make them weekdays:* Choose three consecutive weekdays so that you're truly capturing the amount of movement you typically do.

- *Make them unknown until the end of the day:* Try not to look at your step number until right before you go to bed. Even peeking only every once in a while may cause you to up your pace, whether consciously or unconsciously.

After you have the totals for your three baseline days, add them up and divide that number by three so you know your average baseline steps. Here are guidelines based on your best number of steps:

- *Below 2,500:* Try gradually adding an additional 100 to 200 steps to that total every two to three days.

- *Between 2,501 and 5,000:* Try gradually adding an additional 200 to 400 steps to that total every two to three days.

- *Between 5,001 and 7,499:* Try gradually adding an additional 300 to 500 steps to that total every two to three days.

---

Tip: If you're the type who has your smartphone in your pocket 24/7 (or for at least 90 percent of the day), and your smartphone automatically tracks your steps, and it's turned on right now, you might be able to skip this step altogether. Use an average week from your smartphone's steps log to figure out your baseline number instead. As a bonus, you probably have the most honest estimate since you weren't even aware these steps would be used for this calculation.

---

### Count again—but try a little harder

Once you know your baseline steps, I want you to track your steps again by taking a five-day "boost voyage." I find that this five-day journey is best taken starting on a Monday and continuing through Friday, but because you'll be increasing the number of steps you typically walk, others have found it better to begin on a Wednesday and continue on through Sunday since they may have more time available on the weekend. I leave this entirely up to you.

This time, you'll use the daily average number as a movement motivator to try to increase your daily average in the following order:

- Day 1: Try to walk a minimum of 250 to 500 steps more than your baseline step average
- Day 2: Try to walk a minimum of 500 to 1,000 steps more than your baseline step average
- Day 3: Try to walk a minimum of 750 to 1,500 steps more than your baseline step average
- Day 4: Try to walk a minimum of 1,000 to 2,000 steps more than your baseline step average
- Day 5: Try to walk a minimum of 1,250 to 2,500 steps more than your baseline step average

For example, if your baseline step average was around 3,000, then:

- Day 1: Try walking 3,250 to 3,500 steps
- Day 2: Try walking 3,500 to 4,000 steps
- Day 3: Try walking 3,750 to 4,500 steps
- Day 4: Try walking 4,000 to 5,000 steps
- Day 5: Try walking 4,250 to 5,500 steps

During and after this five-day boost voyage, I want you to listen to your body. Each day, you should always feel challenged *and* comfortable, such that if I asked you to perform that same number of steps the next day, you could do it. Feeling some form of muscle soreness, particularly in your legs, is expected as you may be challenging your muscles beyond what they're used to in an average day. But what I most want you to look out for is fatigue.

- If you continue to feel challenged *and* comfortable, keep increasing your step count each day as prescribed.

- If you find yourself fatigued, then you may have added more steps than your body was ready to handle. If this is the case, return to the number of steps you did the prior day and finish the remainder of the five days walking at that step count.

Your step count at the end of your boost voyage will give you a clear sense of what you're capable of, and *this* is where I want you to start your steps on Day 1 of High Fiber Keto. Now, I don't know the exact number of steps you'll be working with since it will be decided by your individual fitness level. But what I do know is that you need to be true to yourself for your body's sake. You're already putting yourself in a position of moving more—and that's such a powerful step toward giving you an optimized metabolism.

## Do a three-day inactivity audit

Dr. Hausenblas shared that when people write in an activity diary where they map out everything they do during the day, it brings about a stronger sense of awareness.[6] It's the reason that before starting my program, I'd like you to try something similar. But for three straight days, instead of tracking your *activity*, I want you to become more aware of your *inactivity*. You don't need to keep a journal, and I'm not asking you to write anything down if you don't want to. I only want you to go throughout each day and challenge yourself to be aware of two things:

- Every time that you sit
- Every time that you stand in place

Each of these moments of inactivity is an opportunity for moving more, minutely, but no less importantly for your optimized metabolism.

## Set up a series of movement mementos

After you've become aware of the mini moments of metabolic potential at your disposal, during the three days after that, I want you to keep something you can write on and safely stick to things close at hand, such as a pack of sticky notes or a small roll of painter's tape. Every time one of those moments of inactivity emerges, write a reminder to yourself to move and stick it on something where you are, leaving it up until you complete the program. For example, you might do things like these:

- Put a note on your bathroom mirror, in front of the microwave, inside the refrigerator, or anywhere inside your house where you find yourself standing for a few minutes at a time.

- Place a reminder on your computer or TV screen so that you are prompted to stand more instead of staying seated.

- Stick a small piece of tape on the front of your cell phone with the word *move* or *stand* written on it. Or better still, make the word the wallpaper on your phone!

I want you to get creative, because even though I can make suggestions, your daily habits are your own. Regardless of your methodology, I want you to have reminders in place before the program starts. Just do the best you can and remember that you can add more reminders later, even after you begin the program.

## Think of a few subtler signals

Maybe you feel self-conscious about writing little notes to yourself and placing them everywhere. Or you may find that you can't leave reminders in certain places, such as at work, in line at the grocery store, on the sidelines of your child's soccer game, and so forth.

A few people in my trial felt the same way. But surprisingly, they came up with some clever alternatives that allowed them to leave covert reminders to themselves:

- They taped paint chips on their bathroom or kitchen walls. (To others, it simply looked like they were considering a new color option.)

- Some put a colorful decoration that didn't match the decor in rooms where they found themselves the least active. (Every time it caught their eye, it was a silent reminder to move more.)

- Some wore a piece of jewelry—including bracelets, necklaces, and rings—that always needed constant adjusting because they were either too loose or too dangly (Each time they adjusted it, they were reminded that they could be doing something more active at the moment.)

## YOUR PRE-FIX FIBER PLAN

According to Dr. Gershuni and other experts, when you go from eating very little fiber to consuming the appropriate amount, the sudden surge can be quite a surprise to your body and may lead to a few unpleasant gastrointestinal issues, including gas, bloating, constipation, and diarrhea.[7] Even if you eat the average 17 grams daily that most Americans do, getting in that extra 8 to 10 grams to reach the Recommended Daily Allowance (RDA) for fiber can still cause discomfort.[8]

My goal is to prevent those issues and discomforts from happening by helping you to hit the ground running fiber-wise, ready for the changes to come.

### Find your fiber frequency

Similar to your step baseline, it's important to have an understanding of how fiber deficient you may be so that you can prepare your body for the fiber-rich program it's about to enjoy. In order to do this, eat as you usually do for about three to five days and keep track of how many grams of fiber you eat per day. Add up these daily totals, then divide by the number of days involved. The resulting number is your *fiber frequency*, the average amount of fiber you eat daily.

For example, if you eat 10 grams on Monday, 12 grams on Tuesday, 8 grams on Wednesday, and 6 grams on Thursday, that's 36 grams total through the span of 4 days. Divide 36 by 4, and your fiber frequency is 9 grams daily!

- If your fiber frequency is 20 grams or higher: Congratulations! Your body should acclimate to my 22-day program just fine. Continue eating the way you have been right up until you begin the program.

- If your fiber frequency is 10 to 20 grams per day: I want you to incorporate a few specific fiber-rich foods (page 94) into your day for a minimum of 5 days to build your fiber frequency before starting the program

- If your fiber frequency is 9 grams or lower: You'll incorporate a few specific fiber-rich foods (page 94) each day for a minimum of 12 days, depending on how quickly your body adjusts to eating more fiber, to build your fiber frequency before starting the program.

### Glide into becoming fiber fortified

Every expert I interviewed had differing opinions regarding the "perfect" amount or pace for increasing your fiber intake, but all agreed that it's always smart to start slow. As Dr. Gershuni explained, how people respond to fiber is very individualized, so it's always better to ease into seeing how much your body can tolerate before taking it to the next level.

That said, when I compared all the recommendations of how many grams to shoot for and how often to do so, there seems to be a specific range that works better for most people, and that's "3 and 3," meaning, *boost your fiber intake by an additional 3 grams of fiber every three days.*

For example, if you're presently eating 10 grams of fiber, you will raise your fiber frequency to 13 grams for three consecutive days. After three days, you will raise your fiber frequency another 3 grams so that you're eating 16 grams of fiber each day for the next three consecutive days. And so on, until you find yourself at a place where you're eating between 20 and 25 grams of fiber.

But again, everybody's different, which is why Dr. Gershuni believes that introducing more fiber is less of a one-size-fits-all solution and more of a trial-and-error approach.

- If you don't experience any GI issues as you progress, feel free to raise your fiber frequency as recommended. Then keep it at that fiber-fortified level until you start the program.

- If any increase of fiber feels like too much too soon, reduce whatever amount is causing you gastrointestinal discomfort by about 1 to 2 grams and continue to eat that amount daily until your body has acclimated. After that, you can adjust the amount you raise your fiber frequency and increase the number of days to whatever feels best. For example, you can boost it by 2 grams for four days, if you wish, just as long as you continue to build your fiber frequency up to at least 20 grams per day. I want you to move at the pace that works best for you.

**Choose your fiber wisely**

If you are not used to eating a fiber-rich diet, rather than reaping the benefits of fiber, your body may feel uncomfortable with the added digestive nutrients. Bloating, gas, cramps, constipation, loose stool, and intestinal blockage are some of the reactions that can occur. Rather than immediately switching diets, first start with reducing sweet, sugary foods and replacing them with more whole-food options such as fruits and veggies. Try incorporating some of the suggested high-fiber foods in various meals. At least one to two servings of veggies per meal and three servings of fruit per day is recommended, but if this is a major change from your normal eating habits, start with increasing one serving at one meal per day and watch for symptoms. These are just a few options to add into your usual diet:

- An extra serving of green vegetables—the greener they are, the more fiber they generally have. (Note: Cooked vegetables can be easier than raw vegetables in terms of digestion, so feel free to experiment with steaming or roasting them.)

- A handful of berries—raspberries, blackberries, strawberries, blueberries. (If it ends in *berry*, it's full of fiber.)

- Mixing in or sprinkling on some chia seeds or flaxseeds.

- Adding any of the Friendly Fiber choices (page 94) in moderation.

Consider that our hunter-gatherer ancestors ate somewhere around 100 grams of fiber a day. I'm asking you to get your intake up from wherever you are now to a minimum of 20 grams at a rate that you are completely in charge of.

While you may have known the virtues of fiber for human health before, my hope is that you now understand that fiber is the catalyst to optimize your metabolism. Think of fiber as the sun to ketosis's moon—you see, without fiber and enough of it, we miss the magic of how nutritional ketosis can spread vitality throughout your body. Fiber encourages all the beautiful growth of healthy bacteria in your microbiome, which is at the root of your optimized metabolism. By eating the wide variety of fibrous foods and supplements I have laid out for you, your own inner garden of health is bound to bloom. In the next chapter, you'll see just how simple getting the recommended minimum intake of fiber can be.

# SHANNON

### *I felt happier than I had in years.*

Six months ago, I was bigger than I had ever been in my life. I'm guessing it was 185 pounds, but I was so unwilling to step on a scale. My size 10–12 jeans were too tight, but the worst part was that I was in a very toxic relationship for several years that had sent me into a very bad place both emotionally and physically. I was exhausted and sick.

One day, I decided that enough was enough. Maybe it was out of spite that I decided to start taking care of myself when I was constantly being told that I didn't deserve it and couldn't do better. It started off with eating a little less garbage and "treating" myself a little less for doing things that were normal, when I was really just eating to fill the emotional void.

I drank a *ton* of water, but for maybe a week I found that keto was hard. The real changes began when I cut carbs out of my diet. It wasn't that hard at first (the recipes on High Fiber Keto were so good and easy to make). To get through cravings, I focused on how badly I wanted to be healthy again. I felt my energy and mood improve, and I felt absolutely incredible and watched as the pounds fell off.

I was getting compliments as other people started noticing my progress, too. I felt happier than I had in years. I had clarity, focus, and motivation. I am still continuing my journey. I've moved forward from my toxic relationship and am learning how to love myself again in the body I've reclaimed. I am currently studying abroad in Salzburg, Austria, and am proud to report that I climbed a mountain three days ago, a feat that I never dreamed possible for me.

This plan has absolutely changed my life, and I can't wait to face my next adventure head-on.

# CHAPTER NINE

# HIGH FIBER KETO PLAN

## Optimize Your Metabolism: 22-Day Meal and Movement Plan

I have chills.

I have chills because you are about to take the journey that changed me—and one that can also change you.

You have read the science about metabolism, keto, and fiber.

You have learned about all of the foods and nutrients that will transform your body from being a sugar burner to being a fat burner.

You have seen the simple ways you can move more.

You have prepared.

So you are ready to optimize your metabolism. To start living your life with more energy, more vibrancy, and fewer health risks. To experience life-transforming results.

Before you do, I have one request: follow the plan as I have outlined it.

I've laid out my High Fiber Keto plan in a day-by-day format that details exactly what to eat and do diet- and movement-wise each day, while still integrating the personalization for your unique needs that we have already explored. If you follow this plan to the letter, as others before you have, the process of changing over from sugar to fat and ketones—and becoming more metabolically flexible—will happen much faster and take far less effort. While the state of nutritional ketosis may lead to a wide spectrum of health improvements, the factors that allow each of us to get into nutritional ketosis are not universal.

My strategy is for you to begin your process by finding the unique lifestyle and specific carbohydrate tolerance your body requires for nutritional ketosis through first adhering to a strict keto framework, backed by decades of scientific research. Consider these 22 days your own "n of 1" study, where you are both the scientist and the subject. You're going to follow the program with an observant eye and note how you feel and any changes in energy, body composition, sleep, cravings, mood, and, of course, glucose and ketone levels.

By the end of the 22 days, you will have an in-depth understanding of how your personal experience on High Fiber Keto impacts your quality of life and your biochemistry. After that, you can modify your diet, make simple tweaks to the movement plan, or integrate other lifestyle elements to make this plan work even more effectively for your needs.

For example, perhaps your diet feels great, but you realize you're susceptible to stress and need to build in a morning meditation. Or perhaps your workouts need to be adjusted, or maybe you need to really dial in your bedtime routine and improve your sleep hygiene. There are many small changes that you can make in your daily life to yield big results.

## THE OPTIMIZED METABOLISM MEALS

The foods you'll be putting on your plate and pleasuring your palate with go beyond the typical high-fat, low-carb fare required to enter nutritional ketosis. Instead, you'll be sampling some of the most delicious fiber-rich, keto-based meals, snacks, and drinks you've ever tasted that will keep your belly feeling full while making all your good bacteria extremely happy as well.

The specific combinations of meals, drinks, and snacks each day will provide your body with the ideal mix of total electrolytes to help maximize your energy, sleep, hunger, and comfort as your body transforms into a fat burner. The wide diversity of foods and spices offers an additional metabolic boost that makes this program so enjoyable you won't have a desire to cheat. You will be eating the healthiest meals composed by my team of dietitians who used nutritional science to put together all the pieces of the food puzzle properly!

Each group of meals includes the following:

- *Fiber feasts:* The meals you'll be enjoying incorporate specific good fats with different types of fiber to feed your microbiome, improve your metabolism, and help encourage nutritional ketosis.

- *Fat fuel:* Your menu includes Powerphenol-dense smoothies that are a blend of good fats and gut-supportive nutrients. You'll use them either for breakfast or as a snack on the go.

- *Biome boosters:* These tailored meals for lunch and dinner each include a moderate portion of high-quality protein, a source of good fats, nutrient-dense, non-starchy veggies, a serving of fermented food, and polyphenol-rich spices and detoxifying herbs to get your gut and microbiome into nutritional ketosis motion.

- *CraverTamers:* These decadent, high-fat, nutrient-dense keto desserts will satisfy any sweet cravings, supporting your adjustment to nutritional ketosis and promoting metabolic flexibility.

- *MetaBombs metabolism boosters:* These sweet or savory snacks integrate good fats, assorted phytonutrients, prebiotics, probiotic fiber, and other healthy nutrients to enhance your metabolic potential.

# A NOTE ON SODIUM

Sodium is not to be avoided on your High Fiber Keto plan; instead it is one of the plan's most important aspects. As you transition into nutritional ketosis, your body will let go of water because of carb restriction, making hydration and electrolytes incredibly important to preventing dehydration and "keto flu" symptoms.

You'll naturally be getting sodium through the whole foods on your 22-day meal plan, including meat, non-starchy veggies, dairy, and broth, along with the sea salt added in the recipes. Here are some of the sodium superstars:

- 3 ounces canned salmon, 471 mg sodium

- 3 ounces canned sardines, 430 mg sodium

- 1 cup bone broth, 390 mg sodium

- 1 ounce cheddar cheese, 176 mg sodium

- 1 tablespoon sauerkraut, 97 mg sodium

- 1 large egg, 70 mg sodium

- 3 ounces grass-fed beef, 58 mg sodium

- One 5-gram package seaweed snacks, 50 mg sodium

- ¼ cup heavy cream, 30 mg sodium, or 2 tablespoons heavy cream, 15 mg sodium

- 1 stalk celery, 32 mg sodium

When designing these recipes, I included the maximum amount of added salt without sacrificing taste and balance of flavor. However, it can be challenging to meet the recommended 3,000 to 5,000 mg of sodium per day on a keto diet through food alone. We all have different sodium needs based on how fat adapted we are, the climate we live in, how active we are, how much we sweat, our body size, and more.

The first symptoms of low sodium in the blood (hyponatremia) can include headache, nausea, irritability, weakness, drowsiness, palpitations, and low energy. We often attribute these symptoms to "keto flu," but, more accurately, they occur when we aren't getting enough sodium each day. My advice: Dose up as needed. Feel free to adjust the salt in any of the recipes and keep a salt shaker on the table in order to salt your food to taste.

Here are a few of my favorite culinary tricks for adding more sodium to my diet, without necessarily adding more table salt:

- Add 1 to 2 tablespoons of sauerkraut, kimchi, or another fermented vegetable to at least one meal each day.
- Stir 2 teaspoons of miso into a cup of broth or salad dressing.
- Sprinkle powdered seaweed (kelp or dulse) on top of any meal.
- Use milk or cream in place of coconut or almond milk, if dairy is tolerated.

For some, including more salt in the diet requires a shift in mind-set away from dietary rules of the past that shunned salt. But in order to fully embrace the High Fiber Keto lifestyle, you need salt and you will feel so much better with it. As you pay attention to your sodium intake, I encourage you to listen to your body and notice how you feel when you are truly getting enough—the results will astound you!

If you are on a sodium-restricted diet or have concerns about your sodium intake, it's always advisable to talk to your doctor before making any dietary changes.

## THE METABOLISM MOVEMENT CHECKLIST

Each day, you'll see three boxes I want you to check off right before bedtime:

- Did you *Step Up* and reach your daily total? In other words, did you take enough steps?
- Did you *Stand Up* as often as possible? Did you stand more than you sat?
- Did you *Shake Up* as often as possible? Did you move as often as possible when seated?

This portion of the daily planner will help you to reflect on how your day went with regard to reaching your personal movement goal.

Check each box only if you can say that you truly did your best. If for some reason you didn't hit your step count or feel that you could have stood or moved more on any particular day, then leave that box unmarked. But you know what? Don't be discouraged anytime a box is left untouched—it just means that you can do your absolute best the very next day.

## DAY 1

### The Metabolic Meals

**Breakfast:** Mocha Cream Smoothie (page 189)
**Lunch:** Keto Grilled Cheese (page 223)
**Dinner:** Pan-Fried Rosemary Salmon with Sautéed Spinach (page 237)
**Dessert:** Peanut Butter Frozen Yogurt (page 269)
**Snack:** 2 tablespoons coconut butter

### The Metabolic Movements

☐ Did you *Step Up* and reach your daily total?
☐ Did you *Stand Up* as often as possible?
☐ Did you *Shake Up* as often as possible?

**Total calories for the day:** 1,800
**Total percent of calories from fat:** 75%
**Total percent of calories from protein:** 14%
**Total percent of calories from carbs:** 11%
**Total amount of magnesium:** 148 mg
**Total amount of sodium:** 1,041 mg
**Total amount of potassium:** 985 mg

# DAY 2

## The Metabolic Meals

**Breakfast:** Blackberry Yogurt Fiber Bowl (page 192)
**Lunch:** Roast Beef Lettuce Wraps (page 222)
**Dinner:** Meatballs with Zucchini Noodles and Classic Pesto (page 229)
**Dessert:** 1 PB&J Bomb (page 265)
**Snack:** 1 ounce organic cheddar cheese

## The Metabolic Movements

☐ Did you *Step Up* and reach your daily total?
☐ Did you *Stand Up* as often as possible?
☐ Did you *Shake Up* as often as possible?

**Total calories for the day:** 1,820
**Total percent of calories from fat:** 73%
**Total percent of calories from protein:** 17%
**Total percent of calories from carbs:** 10%
**Total amount of magnesium:** 117 mg
**Total amount of sodium:** 1,504 mg
**Total amount of potassium:** 1,142 mg

# DAY 3

## The Metabolic Meals

**Breakfast:** Chia Cinnamon Breakfast Pudding (page 191)
**Lunch:** Deviled Egg Salad (page 199)
**Dinner:** Coconut and Macadamia Nut Chicken with Roasted Green Beans (page 233)
**Dessert:** 1 Pumpkin Pecan Pie Fat Bomb (page 261)
**Snack:** 1 stalk of celery with 1 tablespoon of cream cheese

## The Metabolic Movements

☐ Did you *Step Up* and reach your daily total?
☐ Did you *Stand Up* as often as possible?
☐ Did you *Shake Up* as often as possible?

**Total calories for the day:** 1,910
**Total percent of calories from fat:** 81%
**Total percent of calories from protein:** 10%
**Total percent of calories from carbs:** 9%
**Total amount of magnesium:** 126 mg
**Total amount of sodium:** 507 mg
**Total amount of potassium:** 903 mg

# DAY 4

## The Metabolic Meals

**Breakfast:** Berries and Cream Keto Smoothie (page 190)
**Lunch:** Artichoke and Greens with Grass-Fed Ground Beef (page 202)
**Dinner:** Greens Pesto Chicken (page 234)
**Dessert:** Smoked Salmon Basil Bomb (up to 2) (page 262)
**Snack:** 2 tablespoons pumpkin seeds and 1 tablespoon cacao nibs

## The Metabolic Movements

☐ Did you *Step Up* and reach your daily total?
☐ Did you *Stand Up* as often as possible?
☐ Did you *Shake Up* as often as possible?

**Total calories for the day:** 1,776
**Total percent of calories from fat:** 75%
**Total percent of calories from protein:** 16%
**Total percent of calories from carbs:** 9%
**Total amount of magnesium:** 308 mg
**Total amount of sodium:** 795 mg
**Total amount of potassium:** 1,662 mg

## DAY 5

### The Metabolic Meals

**Breakfast:** Fresh Super Herb, Avocado, and Mozzarella Omelet (page 194)
**Lunch:** Cobb Salad and Keto Crackers (pages 201, 228)
**Dinner:** Grilled Steak with Mashed "Potatoes" (page 235)
**Dessert:** Jalapeño Lime Fat Bomb (up to 2) (page 253)
**Snack:** ½ avocado with a drizzle of olive oil and herbs

### The Metabolic Movements

☐ Did you *Step Up* and reach your daily total?
☐ Did you *Stand Up* as often as possible?
☐ Did you *Shake Up* as often as possible?

**Total calories for the day:** 1,960
**Total percent of calories from fat:** 74%
**Total percent of calories from protein:** 17%
**Total percent of calories from carbs:** 9%
**Total amount of magnesium:** 104 mg
**Total amount of sodium:** 1,274 mg
**Total amount of potassium:** 2,157 mg

## DAY 6

### The Metabolic Meals

**Breakfast:** Chia Cinnamon Breakfast Pudding (page 191)
**Lunch:** Salmon Salad (page 208)
**Dinner:** Turkey Bacon Burger with Creamy Parsley Pesto (page 239)
**Dessert:** Decadent Chocolate Pudding with Raspberries (page 270)
**Snack:** ¼ cup olives

## The Metabolic Movements

- ☐ Did you *Step Up* and reach your daily total?
- ☐ Did you *Stand Up* as often as possible?
- ☐ Did you *Shake Up* as often as possible?

**Total calories for the day:** 1,830
**Total percent of calories from fat:** 75%
**Total percent of calories from protein:** 15%
**Total percent of calories from carbs:** 10%
**Total amount of magnesium:** 162 mg
**Total amount of sodium:** 3,121 mg
**Total amount of potassium:** 1,058 mg

# DAY 7

## The Metabolic Meals

**Breakfast:** Bacon, Spinach, and Cheddar Frittata (page 193)
**Lunch:** Keto Chili (page 219)
**Dinner:** Arugula Salad with Southwest Chicken Strips and
Sautéed Zucchini, drizzled with olive oil (page 268)
**Dessert:** 1 Chocolate Chai Tea Truffle (page 266)
**Snack:** Salmon jerky

## The Metabolic Movements

- ☐ Did you *Step Up* and reach your daily total?
- ☐ Did you *Stand Up* as often as possible?
- ☐ Did you *Shake Up* as often as possible?

**Total calories for the day:** 1,930
**Total percent of calories from fat:** 77%
**Total percent of calories from protein:** 15%
**Total percent of calories from carbs:** 8%
**Total amount of magnesium:** 85 mg
**Total amount of sodium:** 1,137 mg
**Total amount of potassium:** 1,708 mg

# DAY 8

## The Metabolic Meals

**Breakfast:** Blackberry Yogurt Fiber Bowl (page 192)
**Lunch:** Chicken Cabbage Salad with Creamy Hemp Seed
　　Dressing (page 211)
**Dinner:** Flank Steak with Chimichurri Sauce and Baked
　　Spaghetti Squash with Parsley (page 248)
**Dessert:** Smoked Salmon Basil Bomb (up to 2) (page 262)
**Snack:** ¼ cup walnuts

## The Metabolic Movements

☐ Did you *Step Up* and reach your daily total?
☐ Did you *Stand Up* as often as possible?
☐ Did you *Shake Up* as often as possible?

**Total calories for the day:** 1,730
**Total percent of calories from fat:** 74%
**Total percent of calories from protein:** 17%
**Total percent of calories from carbs:** 9%
**Total amount of magnesium:** 161 mg
**Total amount of sodium:** 328 mg
**Total amount of potassium:** 1,226 mg

# DAY 9

## The Metabolic Meals

**Breakfast:** Chia Cinnamon Breakfast Pudding (page 191)
**Lunch:** Mexican Chicken Soup (page 215)
**Dinner:** Chicken Curry with Cauliflower Rice (page 242)
**Dessert:** Maple Walnut Ice Cream (page 267)
**Snack:** 1 hard-boiled egg with sea salt and ½ cup cucumber slices

## The Metabolic Movements

- ☐ Did you *Step Up* and reach your daily total?
- ☐ Did you *Stand Up* as often as possible?
- ☐ Did you *Shake Up* as often as possible?

**Total calories for the day:** 1,920
**Total percent of calories from fat:** 71%
**Total percent of calories from protein:** 18%
**Total percent of calories from carbs:** 11%
**Total amount of magnesium:** 207 mg
**Total amount of sodium:** 483 mg
**Total amount of potassium:** 1,207 mg

## DAY 10

### The Metabolic Meals

**Breakfast:** Berries and Cream Keto Smoothie (page 190)
**Lunch:** Keto BLT (page 225)
**Dinner:** Seared Scallops with Cilantro Mint Sauce (page 241)
**Dessert:** Decadent Chocolate Pudding with Raspberries (page 270)
**Snack:** Easy Slow-Cooker Bone Broth with up to 1 tablespoon
    MCT oil (page 198)

### The Metabolic Movements

- ☐ Did you *Step Up* and reach your daily total?
- ☐ Did you *Stand Up* as often as possible?
- ☐ Did you *Shake Up* as often as possible?

**Total calories for the day:** 1,755
**Total percent of calories from fat:** 79%
**Total percent of calories from protein:** 11%
**Total percent of calories from carbs:** 10%
**Total amount of magnesium:** 274 mg
**Total amount of sodium:** 1,278 mg
**Total amount of potassium:** 1,537 mg

# DAY 11

## The Metabolic Meals

**Breakfast:** Berries and Cream Keto Smoothie (page 190)
**Lunch:** Salmon Caesar Salad with Keto Crackers (pages 205, 228)
**Dinner:** Grass-Fed Burger with Jicama Slaw (page 238)
**Dessert:** Simple Berries and Cream (page 271)
**Snack:** 1 ounce organic cheddar cheese

## The Metabolic Movements

- ☐ Did you *Step Up* and reach your daily total?
- ☐ Did you *Stand Up* as often as possible?
- ☐ Did you *Shake Up* as often as possible?

**Total calories for the day:** 2,005
**Total percent of calories from fat:** 73%
**Total percent of calories from protein:** 16%
**Total percent of calories from carbs:** 11%
**Total amount of magnesium:** 163 mg
**Total amount of sodium:** 801 mg
**Total amount of potassium:** 2,149 mg

# DAY 12

## The Metabolic Meals

**Breakfast:** Blackberry Yogurt Fiber Bowl (page 192)
**Lunch:** Broccoli Cheddar Soup (page 218)
**Dinner:** Keto Bolognese (page 231)
**Dessert:** Pumpkin Pecan Pie Fat Bomb (page 261)
**Snack:** Salmon jerky with 1 cup of tea of choice (suggested: AutophaTea) with up to 1 tablespoon MCT oil

## The Metabolic Movements

- ☐ Did you *Step Up* and reach your daily total?
- ☐ Did you *Stand Up* as often as possible?
- ☐ Did you *Shake Up* as often as possible?

**Total calories for the day:** 1,830
**Total percent of calories from fat:** 74%
**Total percent of calories from protein:** 15%
**Total percent of calories from carbs:** 11%
**Total amount of magnesium:** 75 mg
**Total amount of sodium:** 1,410 mg
**Total amount of potassium:** 565 mg

# DAY 13

## The Metabolic Meals

**Breakfast:** Mocha Cream Smoothie (page 189)
**Lunch:** Spinach, Avocado, and Blueberry Salad (page 212)
**Dinner:** Cauli Mac 'n' Cheese with Steamed Green Beans (page 255)
**Dessert:** Jalapeño Lime Fat Bomb (up to 2) (page 263)
**Snack:** ¼ cup macadamia nuts

## The Metabolic Movements

- ☐ Did you *Step Up* and reach your daily total?
- ☐ Did you *Stand Up* as often as possible?
- ☐ Did you *Shake Up* as often as possible?

**Total calories for the day:** 1,805
**Total percent of calories from fat:** 80%
**Total percent of calories from protein:** 10%
**Total percent of calories from carbs:** 10%
**Total amount of magnesium:** 158.5 mg
**Total amount of sodium:** 1,104 mg
**Total amount of potassium:** 1,071 mg

# DAY 14

## The Metabolic Meals

**Breakfast:** Bacon, Spinach, and Cheddar Frittata (page 193)
**Lunch:** Keto PB&J Sandwich (page 225)
**Dinner:** Fish and Fresh Slaw Tacos with Keto Crackers
(pages 245, 228)
**Dessert:** PB&J Bomb (page 265) with 1 cup of tea of choice
(suggested: AutophaTea) with up to 1 tablespoon MCT oil
**Snack:** Toasted seaweed snacks made with olive oil (5 grams)

## The Metabolic Movements

- ☐ Did you *Step Up* and reach your daily total?
- ☐ Did you *Stand Up* as often as possible?
- ☐ Did you *Shake Up* as often as possible?

**Total calories for the day:** 1,830
**Total percent of calories from fat:** 79%
**Total percent of calories from protein:** 12%
**Total percent of calories from carbs:** 9%
**Total amount of magnesium:** 192 mg
**Total amount of sodium:** 1,106 mg
**Total amount of potassium:** 1,668 mg

# DAY 15

## The Metabolic Meals

**Breakfast:** Chia Cinnamon Breakfast Pudding (page 191)
**Lunch:** Fresh Herb Salad with Wild Salmon with Keto Crackers
(pages 204, 228)
**Dinner:** Beef Stroganoff over Broccoli "Rice" (page 257)
**Dessert:** Decadent Chocolate Pudding with Raspberries (page 270)
**Snack:** 1 cup Easy Slow-Cooker Bone Broth (page 198) with up
to 1 tablespoon MCT oil

## The Metabolic Movements

- ☐ Did you *Step Up* and reach your daily total?
- ☐ Did you *Stand Up* as often as possible?
- ☐ Did you *Shake Up* as often as possible?

**Total calories for the day:** 1,730
**Total percent of calories from fat:** 76%
**Total percent of calories from protein:** 14%
**Total percent of calories from carbs:** 10%
**Total amount of magnesium:** 140 mg
**Total amount of sodium:** 811 mg
**Total amount of potassium:** 1,121 mg

## DAY 16

### The Metabolic Meals

**Breakfast:** Berries and Cream Keto Smoothie (page 190)
**Lunch:** Creamy Curried Chicken Salad Wraps with Keto Crackers (pages 220, 228)
**Dinner:** Peanut Soup with Shrimp (page 232)
**Dessert:** Key Lime Shortbread (page 272)
**Snack:** 1 hard-boiled egg with sea salt and ½ cup cucumber slices

### The Metabolic Movements

- ☐ Did you *Step Up* and reach your daily total?
- ☐ Did you *Stand Up* as often as possible?
- ☐ Did you *Shake Up* as often as possible?

**Total calories for the day:** 1,785
**Total percent of calories from fat:** 72%
**Total percent of calories from protein:** 17%
**Total percent of calories from carbs:** 11%
**Total amount of magnesium:** 102 mg
**Total amount of sodium:** 1,935 mg
**Total amount of potassium:** 1,335 mg

# DAY 17

## The Metabolic Meals

**Breakfast:** Fresh Super Herb, Avocado, and Mozzarella Omelet (page 194)
**Lunch:** Massaged Kale Tahini Salad with Lemon Cauliflower Soup (pages 210, 214)
**Dinner:** Lemon Coconut Chicken with Roasted Broccoli (page 249)
**Dessert:** Peanut Butter Frozen Yogurt (page 269)
**Snack:** ¼ cup walnuts

## The Metabolic Movements

☐ Did you *Step Up* and reach your daily total?
☐ Did you *Stand Up* as often as possible?
☐ Did you *Shake Up* as often as possible?

**Total calories for the day:** 1,925
**Total percent of calories from fat:** 75%
**Total percent of calories from protein:** 16%
**Total percent of calories from carbs:** 9%
**Total amount of magnesium:** 190 mg
**Total amount of sodium:** 919 mg
**Total amount of potassium:** 1,414 mg

# DAY 18

## The Metabolic Meals

**Breakfast:** Blackberry Yogurt Fiber Bowl (page 192)
**Lunch:** Salmon Chowder with Keto Crackers (pages 208, 228)
**Dinner:** Chicken and Waffles (page 246)
**Dessert:** Maple Walnut Ice Cream (page 267)
**Snack:** 1 ounce organic cheddar cheese

## The Metabolic Movements

☐ Did you *Step Up* and reach your daily total?
☐ Did you *Stand Up* as often as possible?
☐ Did you *Shake Up* as often as possible?

**Total calories for the day:** 1,970
**Total percent of calories from fat:** 72%
**Total percent of calories from protein:** 19%
**Total percent of calories from carbs:** 9%
**Total amount of magnesium:** 851 mg
**Total amount of sodium:** 661 mg
**Total amount of potassium:** 493 mg

# DAY 19

## The Metabolic Meals

**Breakfast:** Mocha Cream Smoothie (page 189)
**Lunch:** Avocado Toast (page 227)
**Dinner:** Ground Lamb Patties over Cauliflower Rice with Tzatziki
(page 250)
**Dessert:** 1 Pom Bomb (page 264)
**Snack:** ½ ounce raw almonds

## The Metabolic Movements

☐ Did you *Step Up* and reach your daily total?
☐ Did you *Stand Up* as often as possible?
☐ Did you *Shake Up* as often as possible?

**Total calories for the day:** 1,800
**Total percent of calories from fat:** 78%
**Total percent of calories from protein:** 12%
**Total percent of calories from carbs:** 10%
**Total amount of magnesium:** 201 mg
**Total amount of sodium:** 709 mg
**Total amount of potassium:** 1,468 mg

# DAY 20

## The Metabolic Meals

**Breakfast:** Chia Cinnamon Breakfast Pudding (page 191)
**Lunch:** Greek Salad with Keto Crackers (pages 213, 228)
**Dinner:** Keto Chicken Wings (page 244)
**Dessert:** Jalapeño Lime Fat Bomb (up to 2) (page 263)
**Snack:** 1 to 2 stalks celery topped with 1 tablespoon sunflower seed butter

## The Metabolic Movements

- ☐ Did you *Step Up* and reach your daily total?
- ☐ Did you *Stand Up* as often as possible?
- ☐ Did you *Shake Up* as often as possible?

**Total calories for the day:** 1,820
**Total percent of calories from fat:** 73%
**Total percent of calories from protein:** 16%
**Total percent of calories from carbs:** 11%
**Total amount of magnesium:** 160.5 mg
**Total amount of sodium:** 2,343 mg
**Total amount of potassium:** 943 mg

# DAY 21

## The Metabolic Meals

**Breakfast:** Fresh Super Herb, Avocado, and Mozzarella Omelet (page 194)
**Lunch:** Fresh Green Salad with Poached Eggs and Toasted Pecans and Keto Crackers (pages 209, 228)
**Dinner:** Beef and Mushroom Meatballs over Sautéed Cabbage with Mushroom Cream Sauce (page 253)
**Dessert:** Key Lime Shortbread (page 272)
**Snack:** Toasted seaweed snacks made with olive oil (5 grams)

## The Metabolic Movements

- ☐ Did you *Step Up* and reach your daily total?
- ☐ Did you *Stand Up* as often as possible?
- ☐ Did you *Shake Up* as often as possible?

**Total calories for the day:** 1,855
**Total percent of calories from fat:** 77%
**Total percent of calories from protein:** 17%
**Total percent of calories from carbs:** 6%
**Total amount of magnesium:** 89.53 mg
**Total amount of sodium:** 991 mg
**Total amount of potassium:** 1,136 mg

## DAY 22

### The Metabolic Meals

**Breakfast:** Bacon, Spinach, and Cheddar Frittata (page 193)
**Lunch:** Cauliflower Couscous with Walnuts (page 203) and
Lemon Cauliflower Soup (page 214)
**Dinner:** Parmesan Chicken Tenders with Roasted Brussels
Sprouts (page 258)
**Dessert:** Maple Walnut Ice Cream (page 267)
**Snack:** Easy Slow-Cooker Bone Broth with up to 1 tablespoon
MCT oil (page 198)

### The Metabolic Movements

- ☐ Did you *Step Up* and reach your daily total?
- ☐ Did you *Stand Up* as often as possible?
- ☐ Did you *Shake Up* as often as possible?

**Total calories for the day:** 2,155
**Total percent of calories from fat:** 76%
**Total percent of calories from protein:** 16%
**Total percent of calories from carbs:** 8%

**Total amount of magnesium:** 189 mg
**Total amount of sodium:** 1,001 mg
**Total amount of potassium:** 2,100 mg

When you reach the end of this 22-day journey, you will have learned so much about your body—and I hope you will have felt the changes. The changes in your own energy. The changes in your appetite. The changes in how you feel day to day, hour to hour.

Since I have shifted to a place where my body is utilizing fat instead of sugar as fuel, I have felt all these changes and seen transformations in the markers so important for metabolic health.

Now you're in a perfect position to take what you have learned about yourself and about fat adaptation and make adjustments that work for you. You can experiment with foods and recipes and ingredients to eat what you like best—and with the ratios and amounts that will keep you in nutritional ketosis.

This plan isn't meant to be the end of a "diet." It's meant to be the start of something new.

A new you.

## AMANDA

### *My body and soul are satiated and full.*

I lost both of my parents in their 60s to cancer. And knowing that I was close to that age, I knew I had to do something drastic to keep myself on the planet longer than they had been able to.

My measurements put me in the official "morbidly obese" category—and gave me all of the health issues that go with that unfortunate "title."

So there I was. I love to cook—and apparently eat. And I had to make a choice: bariatric surgery or die an early death. But then keto showed up on my radar.

I didn't want a quick fix. I didn't want to *diet* again. I wanted to cook. I wanted to eat good food. I wanted to be healthy. And I wanted to be here for my son for as long as possible. He has been my biggest supporter and inspiration.

Together, we've been having nightly cooking adventures, and it's been my biggest blessing. We work in the kitchen together making amazing memories and amazing food!

We have created some of the most delicious, fulfilling meals and can't wait to experiment with more. Knowing the recipes are perfectly aligned with our keto lifestyle makes it even more rewarding.

I haven't once looked back, and I'm not even tempted, as my body and soul are both satiated and full. I'm in this for life. Real life! Mission accomplished.

# PART III

# THE
# METABOLISM
# FIX RECIPES

# YOUR GUIDE TO MAXIMIZE YOUR DIET

I'm going to share something with you—and afterward, maybe you'll share something with me.

When I first began to unravel what it would take nutritionally to give someone an optimized metabolism, I wasn't quite sure if it was even remotely possible to create a menu of delicious meals that were ketogenic, rich in fiber, and microbiome-supportive all at the same time—and have each and every one something that seemed familiar.

Your turn—were you wondering the same thing? It's okay if you were because all of that is about to change, just as it did for me.

Like you, I truthfully thought it might require a little compromise. You know, a few sacrifices in terms of taste and texture with at least a handful of recipes—okay, maybe all of them. But then as I began to build out the meals you're about to experience with nutritionists, Ph.D.s, my mother, chefs, and keto influencers, my opinion quickly changed. And let me tell you, I was excited to see that there is absolutely no compromise or sacrifice for the sake of your healthy metabolism. In fact, each recipe is so incredibly tasty, I guarantee you'll forget like I did that the reason you're eating them in the first place is to optimize your metabolism!

## BEFORE YOU START—KNOW YOU CAN SWAP

The longer I've worked in the health and wellness space, the more I've come to understand that one size *never* fits all.

Even though I personally enjoy all the recipes in this book exactly as they are presented, you may need to make a few changes based on your lifestyle or tastes. That's why I designed this quick chart that lets you know what you can substitute if you find that a particular vegetable, fruit, or cut of meat; a certain type of seafood; various forms of dairy or produce; or some random ingredient isn't something you would ordinarily eat.

But in case you're nervous that making a substitution will make a recipe less effective, don't worry. The nutritional information you'll see at the bottom of each recipe may change, but so long as you're following the recipe's measurements and serving sizes, you'll continue to stay in nutritional ketosis, provide your body with plenty of fiber, and enrich your microbiome with the widest variety of pre- and probiotics possible.

Final tip: Even if you have no problem with a recipe the way it's designed, definitely keep the substitutions in mind for more variety. By using them to tweak the recipes the next time around, you can make your meal feel like an entirely different experience—while getting the same metabolism changing results!

| If you don't like this | Then try this | Tips |
|---|---|---|
| **Produce** | | |
| Spinach | Another leafy green such as arugula, chard, or kale | If the spinach is in a cooked dish, choose a heartier green. For salads, mixed greens or lettuce can also be a replacement. |
| Cilantro | Parsley, mint, dill, or another leafy green herb | Interesting aside: Some people have a gene that makes cilantro taste like soap! |
| Cabbage | Kale, brussels sprouts, broccoli, or cauliflower | These vegetables are members of the cruciferous family and contain compounds that support detoxification. |
| Raspberries | Blueberries, blackberries, or strawberries | I want you to substitute one type of berry only for another type of berry because they are perfectly high in fiber and antioxidants—and lower in carbohydrates than other fruits. |
| **Meat** | | |
| Grass-fed beef | Lamb, bison, deer, or elk | Game can be leaner than beef, so try adding an extra tablespoon of fat to the recipe |
| Lamb | Grass-fed beef | Look for grass-fed beef with 85% fat |
| Turkey | Chicken | For both turkey and chicken, choose organic, pasture-raised meat and use bone-in, skin-on cuts. When using ground poultry, always opt for the dark meat for its higher fat and mineral ratios. |

## Seafood

| | | |
|---|---|---|
| Shrimp | Fatty fish such as wild salmon, mackerel, Alaskan cod, or sardines. Or try another seafood such as clams, oysters, or mussels. | Choose smaller fish from cold waters and sustainable seafood. Seafoodwatch.org and ewg.org are good resources. |
| Fish | Another fatty protein, such as grass-fed beef or pastured eggs. | If you have trouble eating fish regularly, consider a daily fish oil supplement such as 1 teaspoon of BioAlaskan fish oil. |
| Canned mackerel | Canned wild salmon or sardines. | Tuna can be high in mercury, so best to eat it no more than 1 to 2 times per month. |

## Dairy

| | | |
|---|---|---|
| Cream or milk | Full-fat coconut milk | The canned coconut milk has a thicker, fattier texture than the boxed or refrigerated options. Choose a BPA-free can. |
| Butter | Ghee, coconut oil, coconut butter, or avocado oil | If you avoid butter because you don't tolerate dairy, ghee may be tolerated and can provide the same healthy fats—minus the dairy proteins. |
| Yogurt | Full-fat coconut yogurt | When choosing plant-based dairy replacements, always look for unsweetened options without any fillers or unnecessary ingredients. |
| Cheese | Replace with nutritional yeast or just omit it from the recipe and replace it with an additional source of fat such as ghee, coconut oil, or olive oil | Nutritional yeast can add a cheesy flavor to savory dishes such as cauliflower mashed potatoes. |

## Eggs

| | | |
|---|---|---|
| Eggs | Another food that has both fat and protein, such as dairy, fish, or chicken (or, for baking, flaxseeds or chia seeds) | 1 tablespoon ground flaxseeds or chia seeds mixed with 3 tablespoons warm water to create a gel can replace 1 egg in a baking recipe. |

| Fermented Foods | | |
|---|---|---|
| Sauerkraut (fermented cabbage) | Another fermented condiment such as kimchi, full-fat yogurt, a dressing made with raw apple cider vinegar, or dill pickles | Look for fermented foods in the refrigerator section of the grocery store. In shelf-stable foods, the beneficial bacteria have been lost during the canning process. |
| **Pantry Items** | | |
| Walnuts | Pecans, macadamia nuts, pili nuts, or pumpkin seeds | Some nuts, such as cashews, are higher in carbs than other choices—so stick with the chosen few I've listed. |
| Coconut aminos | Soy sauce or tamari | Tamari is a gluten-free version of soy sauce. Coconut aminos are a similar condiment that uses coconut nectar instead of soy as the base. |
| Peanuts | Almonds, walnuts, or macadamia nuts | Fun fact: Peanuts are technically a legume (bean) but are much higher in fat and lower in carbs than most legumes and more nutritionally similar to a nut. |
| Coconut milk | Cow or goat milk, or cream | Coconut is a great keto swap for dairy and vice versa! |
| Bone broth | Mineral Broth (page 197) | If drinking a mug of broth isn't your thing, try incorporating it as the liquid in recipes. Collagen is an important protein in bone broth and can also be taken as a protein powder/supplement. |
| Coffee | AutophaTea, black tea, Earl Grey tea with real citrus bergamot, green tea, herbal teas, chicory root coffee replacement, or mushroom coffee replacement such as Four Sigmatic adaptogen blend or Rasa coffee blends. | When choosing decaffeinated options, look for high-quality beans or tea leaves and a water-based decaffeination process. If you're using mushroom coffee, look for blends made with healing mushrooms—for example, reishi, lion's mane, turkey tail, chaga, Cordyceps, shiitake, or maitake. |

Please note: The calories are suggestions, and everyone should take their individual needs into consideration when deciding what to eat. Please consult a medical provider or registered dietitian to customize the meal plan for your personal needs.

Here are some additional notes and considerations to keep in mind as you enjoy the fabulous food over the next 22 days:

- Raw eggs and egg yolks can pose health risks, especially for those with compromised immune systems, including those who are pregnant, young children, and the elderly. Always consult your doctor and make the choice that's best for you.

- Bacon should be nitrite and nitrate free.

- Eggs should be pastured.

- Butter and meats should all be grass-fed or pastured. I recommend 85 percent lean ground beef.

- Choose organic whenever you can!

- All nuts should be raw unless otherwise specified.

- *Pepper* means black pepper unless otherwise specified. For the best taste, I highly recommend always freshly grinding your pepper just before using.

- Pickles and sauerkraut should be traditionally fermented and from the refrigerated section of the grocery store.

- Yogurt should be full fat, plain, and unsweetened.

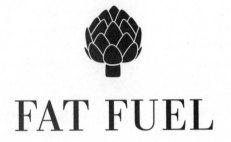

# FAT FUEL

### MOCHA CREAM SMOOTHIE

*Makes 4 servings*

*Prep time: 10 minutes*

I so love this quick and nourishing smoothie on busy mornings. The creaminess of the Greek yogurt and whole-food MCT oil pairs perfectly with the cacao for a rich, chocolaty flavor. The raw cacao powder is also a rich source of antioxidants, which I first fell in love with while working with the Kuna in Panama. The spinach packs a hefty dose of vitamins and minerals without a lot of carbs.

1 cup chilled coffee

2 cups water

2 cups full-fat Greek yogurt

Up to ¼ cup whole-food MCT oil (or coconut oil or butter)

¼ cup raw cacao powder

4 servings collagen powder

2 cups spinach

2 scoops fiber powder

1 cup ice

Place all ingredients in a blender and blend until smooth.

Nutritional analysis per serving (¼ smoothie): calories 330 • fat 25 g • protein 12 g • carbs 19 g • fiber 8 g

## BERRIES AND CREAM KETO SMOOTHIE

*Makes 4 servings*

*Prep time: 10 minutes*

Berries and cream go together like bread and butter (but without the inflammatory impact from the refined flour, of course!). In this keto smoothie, I pair fiber-rich blackberries with silky heavy cream, heart-healthy avocado, and hydrating cucumber to create a delicious smoothie that not only tastes like a decadent treat but indulges your body in the true benefits of the High Fiber Keto lifestyle: long-lasting energy that helps you restore your health and your body one meal at a time. Enjoy this smoothie cold for optimal flavor experience!

1 medium English cucumber (ends removed)

1 avocado

1 cup frozen blackberries

Up to ¼ cup whole-food MCT oil (or coconut butter or oil)

2 scoops fiber powder

1 cup heavy cream

2 cups water

1 cup ice cubes

4 servings collagen powder (optional)

Place ingredients in blender, and blend on high until well mixed, about 30 seconds.

Nutritional analysis per serving (¼ smoothie with collagen powder): calories 455 • fat 41 g • protein 12 g • carbs 17 g • fiber 9 g

# FIBER FEASTS

## CHIA CINNAMON BREAKFAST PUDDING

*Makes 4 servings*

*Prep time: 10 minutes, 8 hours to set*

Chia pudding is a great recipe to make the night before when you're looking for a quick and satisfying breakfast option. The chia seeds and hemp seeds are also both great sources of essential fats and fiber. The reason you'll find Ceylon cinnamon so wonderful—beyond how amazing it tastes—is that it's also rich in polyphenols, which help with blood sugar balance and insulin resistance.[1] It truly is a great supportive spice to add to your diet as you become keto-adapted.

⅔ cup full-fat coconut milk

1⅓ cup macadamia nut milk or water

¼ cup chia seeds

¼ cup hemp seeds

1 to 2 teaspoons monk fruit extract (optional)

2 teaspoons real vanilla extract

2 teaspoons Ceylon cinnamon

¼ teaspoon sea salt

2 scoops fiber powder

4 tablespoons whole-food MCT oil (optional)

**Toppings**

¼ cup pumpkin seeds                    ¼ cup raspberries
¼ cup almonds, chopped              ½ cup full-fat Greek yogurt

Combine the coconut milk, macadamia nut milk or water, chia and hemp seeds, monk fruit extract, vanilla extract, cinnamon, and salt stir until well mixed or blend until combined. Cover and set in the fridge overnight, for at least 8 hours.

The next morning, stir in the fiber and add additional coconut milk until desired consistency is reached.

Serve with toppings and drizzle with MCT oil as desired.

Nutritional analysis per serving (¼ pudding): calories 450 • fat 35 g • protein 12 g • carbs 19 g • fiber 10 g

## BLACKBERRY YOGURT FIBER BOWL

*Makes 4 servings*

*Prep time: 5 minutes*

This fiber-packed yogurt bowl may seem like a decadent combination of incredible tasty ingredients, but there's definitely a metabolic method to its madness. The Greek yogurt provides a nutritious and high-fat base. The walnuts and flaxseed contain alpha-linolenic acid that is essential to get from food (since your body can't make it). Finally, you'll also find blackberries, which are both low in carbohydrates compared with other fruits and high in polyphenol compounds that support metabolism.[2] Put them all together with a hint of fresh mint and you have the perfect way to energize your day!

2 cups full-fat Greek yogurt (or sub full-fat coconut yogurt)
Up to ¼ cup plus 2 tablespoons unsweetened MCT oil powder
4 scoops fiber powder
½ teaspoon monk fruit extract (optional)

## Toppings

¼ cup ground flaxseed

½ cup walnuts

½ cup blackberries

2 tablespoons chopped mint

Up to ¼ cup olive oil

Place the yogurt in a bowl and mix in the MCT oil powder, fiber, and monk fruit extract (if using).

Arrange the toppings over the yogurt, drizzle with olive oil and enjoy immediately.

Nutritional analysis per serving (¼ bowl): calories 370 • fat 28 g • protein 13 g • carbs 21 g • fiber 14 g

# BACON, SPINACH, AND CHEDDAR FRITTATA

*Makes 4 servings*

*Prep time: 10 minutes*

*Cook time: 40 to 50 minutes*

I love making frittatas for breakfast or for company when I'm hosting. Your friends will enjoy them too, even if they're not following a keto lifestyle or interested in optimizing their metabolism—I promise! One reason I relish making these is because eggs are such a complete food, packed with good fats, vitamins, minerals, and carotenoid compounds that give yolks that deep yellow-orange color.

4 slices bacon

4 tablespoons butter or ghee

¼ cup diced onion

8 cups arugula or spinach

½ teaspoon sea salt, divided

8 eggs

4 tablespoons heavy cream or full-fat coconut milk

1 tablespoon chopped fresh oregano or 1½ teaspoons dried oregano

½ cup shredded cheddar cheese (optional)

1 avocado, quartered

Preheat oven to 350° F. In a large skillet over medium heat, cook the 4 pieces of bacon until crispy, flipping halfway through. Remove the bacon from the skillet and allow to cool. Chop or crumble it into smaller pieces.

Add the butter to the skillet with the bacon grease. Add the onions and cook until translucent. Stir in the spinach and ¼ teaspoon of the sea salt and cook until wilted.

In a large bowl, whisk the eggs together with the remaining sea salt and the cream or coconut milk. Mix in the bacon, sautéed onion, spinach, oregano, and cheese.

Pour into a greased cast-iron skillet, place in the oven, and bake until the egg mixture is cooked through, about 35 to 40 minutes. Serve with avocado quarters and sea salt to taste.

Nutritional analysis per serving (¼ frittata): calories 465 • fat 41 g • protein 20 g • carbs 8 g • fiber 4 g

## FRESH SUPER HERB, AVOCADO, AND MOZZARELLA OMELET

*Makes 4 servings*

*Prep time: 10 minutes*

*Cook time: 10 minutes per omelet*

Omelets are such a delicious way to supercharge your metabolism with fresh herbs, which is extremely important for your health. Herbs are not only incredibly low in carbohydrates, but they're packed with health-promoting compounds that target detoxification pathways in the body and help to balance the microbiome.[3]

8 eggs, beaten
½ cup heavy cream
½ teaspoon sea salt
¼ teaspoon pepper
¼ cup butter

2 avocados, thinly sliced
¼ cup chopped cilantro
¼ cup chopped parsley
¼ cup chopped basil
4 ounces shredded cheese, Gouda or mozzarella

Mix eggs with cream, salt, and pepper.

Heat a medium skillet over medium-high heat. Melt ¼ of the butter and tilt the pan to coat the bottom.

Pour in ¼ of the egg mixture.

Gently push the cooked portions from edges toward the center with a spatula so that the uncooked eggs can reach the hot surface. Continue cooking, tilting the pan and gently moving the cooked portions as needed.

When the top surface has thickened and no visible liquid egg remains, place ¼ of the avocado, herbs, and cheese on one side of the omelet; then fold the omelet in half.

When the cheese has melted, remove from heat and slide the omelet onto a plate. Sprinkle with a little sea salt to taste.

Repeat three more times until all omelets are made (or refrigerate remaining mixture to save it for future use).

Nutritional analysis per serving (1 omelet): calories 480 • fat 40 g • protein 23 g • carbs 4 g • fiber 5 g

# 'BIOME BOOSTERS

### MINERAL BROTH (VEGAN)

*Makes 24 servings*

*Prep time: 10 minutes*

*Cook time: 2 to 4 hours*

Broth is such an important staple on a ketogenic diet and a terrific source of minerals, particularly electrolytes that really help you make a comfortable transition from being a sugar burner to being a fat burner. This broth draws its minerals from vegetables and includes celery, which is particularly high in sodium and important for your metabolism while following keto, along with a few trace minerals (such as iodine) that come from the seaweed. I love sipping on a mug of broth as a snack, but I also enjoy including it in my cooking as a flavor upgrade from water.

2 carrots

2 leeks

4 garlic cloves, smashed

4 ounces shiitake mushrooms

1 bunch of celery

1-inch piece of ginger, sliced

½ bunch of parsley

⅛-inch strip of kombu seaweed

2 bay leaves

1 teaspoon black peppercorns

1 tablespoon sea salt or more to taste

Wash the vegetables and cut them to fit into a large stockpot.

Place all ingredients in a large stockpot, cover with water, and bring to a boil.

Reduce heat and simmer for up to 4 hours.

Strain the broth and store in glass containers in the fridge (for 3 to 4 days) or in the freezer (for up to 6 months).

Nutritional analysis per serving (1 cup): calories 30 • fat 2 g • protein 7 g • carbs 2 g • fiber 0 g

## EASY SLOW-COOKER BONE BROTH

*Makes 16 servings*

*Prep time: 10 minutes*

*Cook time: 8 hours*

Not only is this nourishing bone broth rich in minerals, but it's also a top source of collagen protein that supports digestion and nourishes both your hair and skin. It's even good for your brain: chicken broth seems to improve both working and short-term memory in adults.[1] Adding raw apple cider vinegar to the broth really helps to draw out the minerals, such as calcium and collagen, from the bones and into the broth.

Bones from 1 small organic chicken or the whole chicken or 2 pounds of beef bones

2 carrots, coarsely chopped

2 stalks of celery, coarsely chopped

1 small onion, coarsely chopped (can be left unpeeled)

2 garlic cloves (can be left whole and unpeeled)

1 tablespoon raw apple cider vinegar

1 tablespoon sea salt (or more to taste)

Place bones or chicken in a large (6 quart) slow cooker.* Add carrots, celery, onion, garlic, and vinegar. Fill slow cooker with enough water to cover the chicken and vegetables, leaving 1 to 2 inches of space at the top so the broth doesn't overflow.

Cook on low throughout the day for about 8 hours. Stir in sea salt, taste and add more to taste.

Turn the heat off and when cool enough, strain the broth, and store in the fridge or freezer.

*If you only have a smaller slow cooker, you can use the amount of bones or chicken pieces that will fit.

Nutritional analysis per serving (1 cup): calories 30 • fat 2 g • protein 7 g • carbs 2 g • fiber 0 g

## DEVILED EGG SALAD

*Makes 4 servings*

*Prep time: 15 minutes*

Deviled eggs are not just for party trays anymore. When you upgrade this classic appetizer with good fats from avocado oil and serve it with a low-carb salad with fresh veggies, herbs, and fermented pickles— well now, you're steering yourself toward optimal health!

Tip: I mentioned this in the "swap section" at the beginning of this chapter, but when choosing pickles, look for ones in the refrigerated section of the store that don't contain any added sugar. If they have been canned to be shelf-stable, you'll miss out on the benefits of the natural probiotics present in the traditionally fermented versions.[2]

### Deviled Eggs

4 eggs, hard-boiled

⅓ cup Avocado Mayo (page 200)

2 tablespoons chopped pickles

Paprika, for garnish

4 cups arugula or spinach

½ teaspoon sea salt (or more to taste), divided

A few sprigs of dill or chives, finely chopped, for garnish

½ large cucumber, sliced

⅓ cup cherry tomatoes, halved

1 avocado, sliced

Olive oil (to taste)

Carefully slice each egg in half lengthwise and remove the yolk. Place the yolks in a bowl and mix with Avocado Mayo.

Spoon half the mixture back into each egg half and top with pickles, a sprinkle of paprika, ¼ teaspoon sea salt per egg, and fresh chives. Toss greens, cucumber, and tomatoes with olive oil.

Place 1 cup of greens mixture on each plate and top with 2 deviled egg halves.

Sprinkle a generous amount of sea salt over eggs and salad.

Place ¼ of the sliced avocado around each salad.

Nutritional analysis per serving (2 egg halves with green salad and sliced avocado): calories 580 • fat 63 g • protein 9 g • carbs 6 g • fiber 3 g

### Avocado Mayo

*Makes about 1 cup*

I learned how to make mayonnaise from my grandfather in France, and this updated version with avocado oil is perfect for your High Fiber Keto plan, as you'll see from its use throughout the recipes. It is quite simple to make and such an easy way to add good-quality fats from the egg yolks and avocado oil to your salads, sandwiches, and dips. In fact, my kids often dip their veggies directly into the fresh batch of mayo!

1 egg

1 egg yolk

1½ teaspoons Dijon mustard

1½ tablespoons lemon juice

¾ teaspoon sea salt (or more to taste), divided

½ teaspoon turmeric

¾ cup avocado oil

Place the egg and egg yolk, mustard, lemon juice, salt, and turmeric in a food processor.

Process until combined (about 30 seconds). Then with the food processor running, use the attachment that allows you to slowly add oil to add the avocado oil, blending until it is completely emulsified.

Taste for salt, adding more if preferred. Store mayo in the refrigerator.

## COBB SALAD

*Makes 4 servings*

*Prep time: 10 minutes*

Cobb salads that you order in any restaurant may technically be keto, but they typically don't use high-quality fats or proteins, and this can turn the meal into something that triggers an inflammatory response.[3] Since one of my goals for you on your metabolic journey is to reduce inflammation, I've upgraded the Cobb to include only the highest quality versions of this traditional salad's ingredients, plus added some extra nutrition from broccoli sprouts and sunflower seeds!

1 head romaine lettuce, coarsely chopped

8 slices bacon, cooked

4 eggs, hard-boiled and chopped

¼ cup sunflower seeds

2 cups shredded cabbage

1 cup chopped parsley

1 cup broccoli sprouts

¼ cup plus 2 tablespoons olive oil or avocado oil

2 tablespoons lemon juice

1 teaspoon raw apple cider vinegar

½ teaspoon sea salt

Pepper to taste

1 avocado, quartered

Place lettuce, bacon, eggs, sunflower seeds, cabbage, parsley, and broccoli sprouts into a large bowl.

Drizzle with olive oil, lemon juice, and vinegar. Add salt and pepper. Toss to combine, and top with avocado. Serve cold with another sprinkle of sea salt to taste.

Nutritional analysis per serving (¼ salad): calories 470 • fat 40 g • protein 16 g • carbs 16 g • fiber 9 g

## ARTICHOKE AND GREENS WITH GRASS-FED GROUND BEEF

*Makes 4 servings*

*Prep time: 10 minutes*

Artichokes are one of my favorite foods! They're delicious, of course, but what often goes ignored is how they're also packed with so much fiber and prebiotics that they're a feast for all the beneficial bacteria in your gut microbiome.[4] This unappreciated veggie is also sulfur-rich, which helps to support the detoxification that occurs as your body transitions into nutritional ketosis. I try to add artichokes to my diet whenever I can, and I hope you will too!

Note: You can easily make the ground meat ahead of time or substitute the meat for canned sardines, salmon, or clams, for both convenience and added nutrition. These alternate options supply omega-3 fatty acids and protein, both of which fuel your body while on High Fiber Keto. Look for lightly smoked sardines with bones or salmon with skin and bones to provide you a boost in calcium. Add a little fresh sea salt to bring out the natural salty and savory flavor.

1 tablespoon avocado oil

8 ounces ground grass-fed beef

8 cups mixed greens

2 cups chopped parsley

10 artichoke hearts (canned, or cooked from frozen)

½ cup pumpkin seeds

¼ cup broccoli sprouts

¼ cup olive oil

1 teaspoon lemon juice

2 teaspoons raw apple cider vinegar

½ teaspoon sea salt

Pepper to taste

1 avocado, sliced

2 tablespoons olive oil, plus more to drizzle before serving

Heat a skillet over medium heat. Add 1 tablespoon avocado oil and the beef. Break up the beef and stir occasionally until cooked through.

While the beef is cooking, place mixed greens, parsley, artichoke hearts, pumpkin seeds, and broccoli sprouts in a medium sized bowl.

Toss with olive oil, lemon juice, vinegar, salt, and pepper.

Top with the ground beef, avocado, and additional olive oil, and sprinkle with a little extra sea salt and lemon juice, if desired. Serve immediately.

Nutritional analysis per serving (¼ salad): calories 495 • fat 40 g • protein 22 g • carbs 14 g • fiber 6 g

## CAULIFLOWER COUSCOUS WITH WALNUTS

*Makes 4 servings*

*Prep time: 5 minutes*

*Cook time: 10 minutes*

This salad is the perfect example of a comforting grainlike salad with fresh herbs and a rich dressing. Enjoy the creativity of cooking with keto as you learn to substitute cauliflower for rice, potatoes, or even couscous! The best part about being in a state of nutritional ketosis is that I find I no longer miss those starchy foods. In fact, I tend to like the cauliflower version more than actual couscous for the delicious flavor and nutritional benefits.[5]

¼ cup ghee or butter

4 cups packaged riced cauliflower (frozen or fresh)

½ teaspoon cumin seeds

½ cup Mineral Broth (page 197)

¼ cup almonds, finely chopped

1 cup chopped cilantro

1 cup chopped parsley

½ teaspoon sea salt

Pepper to taste

½ cup walnuts

1 cup sauerkraut

Heat ghee in medium saucepan pan over medium-high heat.

Add cauliflower and cumin seeds and stir until they become fragrant and start to brown (about 2 minutes). Note: If using frozen cauliflower rice, cook the rice over medium heat about 3 to 5 minutes and then add the cumin seeds.

Add the broth carefully (it will spatter and pop) and bring to a boil. Reduce heat, cover, and simmer until the cauliflower is tender (about 5 minutes).

Remove from heat and allow to cool a few minutes; then fluff with a fork.

Mix in almonds, cilantro, parsley, salt, and pepper, and top with walnuts.

Serve with a side of sauerkraut and an extra sprinkle of sea salt to taste.

Nutritional analysis per serving (¼ couscous): calories 420 • fat 38 g • protein 10 g • carbs 14 g • fiber 7 g

## FRESH HERB SALAD WITH WILD SALMON

*Makes 4 servings*

*Prep time: 10 minutes*

Wild salmon is a fatty fish that's very high in the anti-inflammatory omega-3 fat EPA and tends to be on the list of low-mercury fish,[6] so it always has my vote. I also love the ease of using canned fish and then mixing it with fresh herbs, veggies, and some lime juice to create a filling—and fast and easy to make—weekday salad.

Note: If you already love wild salmon and are feeling adventurous, I'd like you to try mackerel since it is one of the top five healthiest and lowest fish in mercury. It supplies omega-3 fatty acids and protein, both of which fuel your body while on High Fiber Keto. Add a little fresh sea salt to bring out the natural salty and buttery flavor. However, if you truly don't like salmon or mackerel, you can substitute 2 ounces dark meat turkey (roasted, baked, or slow cooked).

8 cups mixed greens

2 cups shredded cabbage

¼ cup chopped dill

¼ cup chopped basil

¼ cup chopped cilantro

4 ounces feta cheese, cubed (optional)

⅓ cup olive oil

4 teaspoons lime juice

½ teaspoon sea salt

Pepper to taste

2 cans wild salmon in olive oil

1 cup sauerkraut

Mix salad greens, cabbage, dill, basil, cilantro, and feta (if using) in a bowl.

Toss with oil, lime juice, salt, and pepper.

Top with wild salmon, sprinkle some sea salt over the fish, and serve with a side of sauerkraut.

Nutritional analysis per serving (¼ salad): calories 385 • fat 35 g • protein 15 g • carbs 7 g • fiber 1 g

## SALMON CAESAR SALAD

*Makes 4 servings*

*Prep time: 15 minutes*

*Cook time: 8 minutes*

My take on the classic Caesar salad is packed full of good fats from literally every direction, including the egg yolks, anchovies, Greek yogurt, and salmon. The dressing may be my favorite part, though, because it's so creamy and comforting. But what really takes the nutrition up a notch are the spinach and broccoli sprouts mixed in. I think you'll be coming back to this combination over and over again!

### Dressing
*Makes about 1¼ cup*

2 egg yolks

½ teaspoon sea salt

Dash of pepper

6 garlic cloves, chopped

4 anchovy fillets

4 teaspoons Dijon mustard

¼ cup lemon juice

2 tablespoons full-fat Greek yogurt

1 cup avocado oil

## Salad

2 tablespoons avocado oil

Four 4-ounce wild Alaskan salmon fillets

½ teaspoon sea salt, divided

2 heads romaine lettuce, coarsely chopped

4 cups spinach

½ cup broccoli sprouts

¼ cup shredded Parmesan cheese

Make the dressing: Add egg yolks, salt, pepper, garlic, and anchovies to a blender. Blend until combined, about 15 seconds. Add mustard, lemon juice, and yogurt and blend again. With the blender still running, carefully remove the blender top and slowly pour in the oil until the dressing is emulsified. Set aside.

Cook the fish: Heat a large, heavy skillet (cast iron if you have it) over medium heat and then add the oil. Place salmon fillets skin side down in the skillet and increase the heat to high. Cook for 3 minutes, sprinkle with salt, and turn the salmon over. Cook for 5 minutes or until browned. Don't overcook; salmon is done when it easily flakes with a fork. Remove from the pan, sprinkle with a little more salt, and set aside.

Place the lettuce, spinach, and broccoli sprouts in a medium bowl. Spoon ¼ cup or more of the dressing onto the salad and toss to combine. Add the Parmesan cheese and top the salad with the seared salmon.

Nutritional analysis per serving (¼ salad): calories 450 • fat 32 g • protein 33 g • carbs 7 g • fiber 4 g

## SUPERFOOD BLT BOWL

*Makes 4 servings*

*Prep time: 10 minutes*

*Cook time: 6 minutes*

In this particular salad, I replaced lettuce with finely chopped kale,[7] which I find has such a lovely texture and flavor when the dressing has been massaged into it! After it's topped with bacon and you've tasted how delicious it is, you will never again look at salad and think, *How boring.*

Tip: When choosing bacon for this dish, look for pasture-raised or organic versions with minimal amounts of added sugar.

¼ cup balsamic vinegar

¼ cup olive oil

2 tablespoons Dijon mustard

½ teaspoon sea salt

½ teaspoon pepper

8 ounces bacon

4 cups kale, finely chopped

1 cup cherry tomatoes, halved

½ cup sunflower seeds

1 cup broccoli sprouts

1 avocado, chopped

½ cup traditionally fermented pickles, diced

Mix the vinegar, oil, mustard, salt, and pepper in a small bowl with a whisk or a fork to combine well. Set aside.

Heat a medium pan over high heat. Add the bacon and cook on each side approximately 3 minutes or until crispy, or it reaches your desired level of doneness. Place the bacon on a plate lined with a paper towel to soak up extra oil.

Combine the kale and dressing in a large bowl and with clean hands massage the kale to make sure the dressing coats it well. Add the cherry tomatoes and sunflower seeds and toss to combine. Top with most of the broccoli sprouts, the avocado, and the pickles.

Chop the bacon into small pieces, sprinkle it over the salad, and top with the remaining fresh sprouts.

Nutritional analysis per serving (¼ bowl): calories 410 • fat 34 g • protein 15 g • carbs 16 g • fiber 6 g

## SALMON SALAD

*Makes 4 servings*

*Prep time: 10 minutes*

Tahini (which is made from ground sesame seeds) is so creamy and flavorful in this salad dressing, and it pairs perfectly with the salmon and watercress. Tip: If you haven't tried watercress before, it's often sold with the roots attached. It's those roots that make it so nourishing because they pull a lot of minerals from the soil, so when you can purchase with the roots on, please do. Before use, discard the roots and eat the leaves. Watercress is also a cruciferous vegetable, which means it is highly detoxifying.[8] But beyond its many health benefits, I just love this green for its peppery flavor, and I use it wherever possible, including in salads like this one, as a fresh component to cooked meals, and even blended up as part of a pesto.

Two 5-ounce cans wild Alaskan salmon (sockeye salmon with skin and bones)

¼ cup Avocado Mayo (page 200)

¼ cup tahini

Juice of ½ fresh lemon

2 teaspoons raw apple cider vinegar

½ cup celery, chopped

1 teaspoon turmeric

½ teaspoon sea salt

Pepper to taste

Lettuce leaves (optional)

Mixed greens (optional)

2 cups watercress (optional)

¼ cup olive oil, plus more to drizzle before serving (optional)

Open and drain the salmon.

Combine the salmon, Avocado Mayo, tahini, lemon juice, vinegar, celery, turmeric, sea salt, and pepper in a bowl. Use a fork to mix well.

Optional: Serve salmon salad in a lettuce wrap or over a large plate of mixed greens. Top with watercress. Drizzle salad with olive oil as desired.

Nutritional analysis per serving (¼ salad): calories 430 • fat 38 g • protein 21 g • carbs 5 g • fiber 1 g

# FRESH GREEN SALAD WITH POACHED EGGS AND TOASTED PECANS

*Makes 4 servings*

*Prep time: 10 minutes*

I find that simple recipes can really highlight the flavors of certain ingredients—and that's exactly what I love about this one. Dandelion leaves are a food I have been incorporating for quite some time after my wise grandmother (affectionately known as my Mutti) introduced me to their versatility. They stimulate digestion and support the liver, and they're even rich in prebiotic fiber to balance the microbiome.[9] Combining them with some simple mixed greens and herbs, then topping it all with a runny egg ever so slightly mutes their bitterness to make a well-balanced salad that tastes good as it heals you!

4 cups mixed greens

4 cups chopped dandelion leaves (or arugula or another bitter green)

2 cups parsley

½ cup olive oil

2 tablespoons raw apple cider vinegar

½ teaspoon sea salt

Pepper to taste

8 poached eggs

¼ cup pecans, lightly roasted

Place the mixed greens, dandelion leaves, and parsley in a bowl and add the oil and vinegar.

Sprinkle with the salt and add pepper to taste.

Divide into 4 bowls. Top each bowl with 2 poached eggs and 1 tablespoon pecans.

Nutritional analysis per serving (¼ salad): calories 370 • fat 33 g • protein 14 g • carbs 6 g • fiber 2 g

## MASSAGED KALE TAHINI SALAD

*Makes 4 servings*

*Prep time: 10 minutes*

I truly believe that cooking is therapeutic and helps to build a healthy relationship with food, and there's research to support this.[10] When I'm in the kitchen, I like to use all of my senses, including touch—and this recipe always lets me do just that. It turns out that massaging kale with your hands actually helps to break down its cell walls, which releases water and tenderizes the kale—it's quite frankly one of my most beloved kitchen hacks.

2 bunches of kale, de-stemmed and chopped

½ teaspoon sea salt

1 cucumber, chopped

⅓ cup tahini

2 tablespoons olive oil

2 teaspoons raw apple cider vinegar

2 garlic cloves, finely chopped

¼ chopped cup mint

¼ cup hemp seeds

Place the kale in a bowl with the sea salt. Massage the kale with your hands for a few minutes until it starts to wilt. Set aside for a few minutes.

Add the cucumber, tahini, oil, and vinegar to the bowl. Mix until tahini is thoroughly combined.

Add the garlic, mint, and hemp seeds and mix everything together. Taste and add salt if desired.

Nutritional analysis per serving (¼ salad): calories 310 • fat 24 g • protein 12 g • carbs 15 g • fiber 10 g

# CHICKEN CABBAGE SALAD WITH CREAMY HEMP SEED DRESSING

*Makes 4 servings*

*Prep time: 10 minutes*

*Cook time: 15 minutes*

One of my favorite ways to make a creamy, satisfying salad dressing is to blend whole nuts or seeds into it. This recipe features the incredible hemp seed, rich in omega-3 fats, protein, and fiber! The nutty and savory flavor mixes perfectly with this hearty salad. Hemp seeds are a great source of minerals, including the important mineral electrolytes of magnesium, potassium, calcium, and sodium.[11]

2 tablespoons coconut oil

12 ounces chicken thighs, cut into 1-inch cubes

½ teaspoon plus up to ¼ teaspoon sea salt and pepper to taste

½ teaspoon paprika

4 tablespoons olive oil plus up to 4 additional tablespoons (optional)

1 teaspoon lime juice

1 teaspoon raw apple cider vinegar

¼ cup hemp seeds

¼ cup fresh parsley

1 head green cabbage, thinly sliced (about 4 cups)

4 cups arugula

2 scallions, thinly sliced

¼ cup cashew pieces

Heat a large skillet on medium-high heat and add coconut oil.

In a bowl, toss the chicken with ½ teaspoon sea salt, pepper, and paprika and add to the hot skillet.

Arrange the chicken in a single layer and cook until golden brown, flipping to cook each side until cooked thoroughly and golden.

In a blender, combine the olive oil, lime juice, vinegar, hemp seeds, parsley, and remaining salt and pepper. Blend until smooth, adding water, if needed, to achieve a creamy consistency.

Toss the cabbage, arugula, and scallions in the dressing and divide between 4 bowls. Top with the chicken and cashews.

Nutritional analysis per serving (¼ salad): calories 580 • fat 47 g • protein 30 g • carbs 7 g • fiber 3 g

# SPINACH, AVOCADO, AND BLUEBERRY SALAD

*Makes 4 servings*

*Prep time: 10 minutes*

I grew up on a biodynamic farm, and this is the type of meal we would often eat after picking greens and herbs from the garden. This simple salad delights with a pop of flavor that's hard to describe—but definitely delicious! What I really love about this meal is the addition of wild blueberries, which are smaller yet much higher in polyphenols[12] than the cultivated blueberries most people buy in the store. Tip: If you can't find fresh wild blueberries, you can always substitute frozen or any fresh organic blueberries you might find locally.

3 cups spinach

1 cup cilantro

2 avocados, quartered

½ cup wild blueberries

¼ cup hemp seeds

1 tablespoon lemon juice

4 tablespoons olive oil, plus more to drizzle before serving (optional)

½ teaspoon sea salt

Pepper to taste

¼ cup macadamia nuts, chopped

Place the spinach, cilantro, avocado, blueberries, and hemp seeds into a bowl.

Drizzle the lemon juice and oil over the salad.

Season with salt and pepper and toss.

Divide the salad among 4 bowls and serve topped with the macadamia nuts and additional olive oil as desired.

Nutritional analysis per serving (¼ salad): calories 470 • fat 48 g • protein 6 g • carbs 9 g • fiber 4 g

## BONUS SALAD: GREEK SALAD

*Makes 4 servings*

*Prep time: 15 minutes*

This salad isn't in the High Fiber Keto meal plan—it's a bonus that you can enjoy after the 22 days are over or as a substitute for another salad, if you prefer. Its classic combination of cucumber, tomato, feta cheese, and olives always reminds me of Greece! Personally, when I pack this salad for lunch, I like to combine all of the ingredients *except* the greens, and then mix in the greens just before I'm ready to eat it. I love how all of the flavors blend together, and I think you'll love it as much as I do.

1 head romaine lettuce, chopped

2 cups spinach

¼ small red onion, thinly sliced

1 cup pitted black or green olives, halved

½ green bell pepper, chopped

1 tomato, chopped

1 small cucumber, sliced into half-moons

2 ounces full-fat feta cheese crumbles

1 cup chopped parsley

4 tablespoons olive oil

2 tablespoons full-fat Greek yogurt

1 teaspoon dried oregano

1 tablespoon raw apple cider vinegar

1 teaspoon lemon juice

1 tablespoon Parmesan cheese

¼ teaspoon sea salt

Pepper to taste

12 ounces grilled skin-on chicken thighs

Combine the lettuce, spinach, onion, olives, bell pepper, tomato, cucumber, feta, and parsley in a large bowl.

In a separate bowl, whisk together the olive oil, yogurt, oregano, vinegar, lemon juice, and Parmesan.

Pour the dressing over the salad, toss, and season the salad with salt and pepper. Taste and add additional salt if necessary.

Place the grilled chicken on top and serve.

Nutritional analysis per serving (¼ salad): calories 520 • fat 40 g • protein 27 g • carbs 14 g • fiber 3 g

## LEMON CAULIFLOWER SOUP

*Makes 4 servings*

*Prep time: 10 minutes*

*Cook time: 45 minutes*

Soups are such a great way to include nourishing broths in your diet, as well as retain ascorbic acid and other antioxidants that typically get lost when you steam veggies.[13] But that's not the only reason I adore this recipe. This cauliflower soup is creamy, comforting, and incredibly adaptable if you don't eat dairy. Simply use the coconut cream and the coconut yogurt instead of the dairy and omit the sprinkle of Parmesan cheese, perhaps sprinkling on a little nutritional yeast instead. For a vegan version, you can substitute Mineral Broth (page 197) for the Easy Slow-Cooker Bone Broth if you like. But no matter how you tailor it, every variety is full of flavor and equally wonderful!

¼ cup olive oil, divided

1 medium onion, finely chopped

2 cloves garlic, minced

3 cups Easy Slow-Cooker Bone Broth (page 198)

4 cups cauliflower florets

1 teaspoon sea salt

1 tablespoon fresh dill or ½ teaspoon dried dill

2 tablespoons fresh lemon juice

½ cup heavy cream or coconut cream

1 tablespoon Parmesan cheese

2 tablespoons full-fat Greek yogurt

Add the oil to a large pot and heat over medium heat. Add the onion and cook for about 5 minutes. Add the garlic and continue to cook until the onions are translucent, about 3 more minutes, being careful to not let the garlic burn.

Add the broth and bring to a low boil. Add the cauliflower, salt, and dill and return to a boil. Reduce to a simmer and cook for 20 to 30 minutes or until you can easily pierce the cauliflower with a fork; then remove from heat.

Using an immersion blender, blend the soup until smooth. Use a metal mesh sieve to strain the soup into a large bowl. Use caution when transferring hot liquid.

Pour the strained soup back into the pot over medium heat. Add the lemon juice, cream, and Parmesan cheese, and heat until hot all the way through (about 1 to 2 minutes).

Serve immediately topped with the yogurt.

Nutritional analysis per serving (¼ soup): calories 310 • fat 28 g • protein 11 g • carbs 10 g • fiber 3 g

## MEXICAN CHICKEN SOUP

*Makes 4 servings*

*Prep time: 15 minutes*

*Cook time: 50 minutes*

Spicy and savory, this soup will be a home run for your whole family, and I say that from experience, because that's exactly what it is for mine! My kids have so much fun putting their own toppings on this soup that they're not even aware of how I'm getting nourishing fats and broth into their diet. Tip: Do your metabolism a favor and make extra to freeze for a quick work lunch or weeknight dinner.

2 tablespoons avocado oil, divided

1 pound bone-in skinless chicken thighs, cubed

½ small white onion, diced

3 cloves garlic, diced

½ green bell pepper, diced

1 tablespoon chili powder

1 teaspoon dried oregano

¾ teaspoon sea salt

½ teaspoon pepper

2 tablespoons lime juice

1 medium tomato, diced

3 cups Easy Slow-Cooker Bone Broth (page 198)

1 cup heavy cream or full-fat coconut milk

**Toppings**

| | |
|---|---|
| Chopped cilantro | Avocado |
| Shredded cheddar cheese | Black olives |
| Sour cream | |

Add 1 tablespoon of the oil and all of the chicken to a heavy stockpot over medium heat. Sauté until the chicken is browned on each side and cooked through, about 10 minutes. Remove the chicken and set aside.

Add the second tablespoon of avocado oil to the pot. Add the onion and sauté until translucent, about 3 to 4 minutes. Add the garlic and bell pepper and sauté a couple minutes more.

Add the chili powder, oregano, salt, pepper, lime juice, tomato, and broth. Stir and let the soup come to a boil. Reduce the heat, cover, and let it simmer for about 25 minutes. Add the cooked chicken and continue simmering for 10 minutes more.

Turn off the heat and stir in the cream.

Serve the soup hot with your favorite keto toppings.

Nutritional analysis per serving (¼ soup): calories 470 • fat 32 g • protein 32 g • carbs 10 g • fiber 4 g

## SALMON CHOWDER

*Makes 4 servings*

*Prep time: 15 minutes*

*Cook time: 50 minutes*

Wild salmon is one of my favorite foods because of how rich it is in omega-3 fats[14] that are anti-inflammatory, are important for brain health, and help your skin glow.[15] Because of all those benefits, I include it in my diet in a range of ways: fresh, canned, smoked, and even as you're about to enjoy—in a chowder! This particular recipe is just so rich and decadent that if you're the type who finds fish boring, your taste buds will change their opinion about salmon soon, I promise!

2 tablespoons coconut oil

1 small onion, chopped

3 cloves garlic, minced

1 small head cauliflower, cut into bite-sized florets

3 stalks celery, chopped

4 cups Mineral Broth (page 197)

1 tablespoon raw apple cider vinegar

1 tablespoon chopped thyme

1 tablespoon chopped dill

1 teaspoon sea salt

1-pound salmon fillet, cut into bite-sized pieces

One 15-ounce can full-fat coconut milk

2 tablespoons lemon juice

¼ cup chopped parsley

Melt the oil in a large pot over medium heat. Sauté the onion until soft and translucent, about 5 minutes. Add the garlic and cook another minute.

Stir in the cauliflower and celery. Cook for another 5 to 10 minutes. Stir in the broth, vinegar, thyme, dill, and salt. Reduce the heat, cover, and simmer for 30 minutes, until the vegetables soften.

Carefully place 2 cups of the soup into a blender to puree, taking out the center of the lid and covering the opening with a dish towel to avoid a buildup of pressure from the heat, and then add the puree back into the soup pot. (Or use an immersion blender and partially puree the soup in the pot.)

Add the salmon and coconut milk and continue to simmer until the fish is cooked.

Remove from the heat and stir in the lemon juice. Garnish with the parsley and serve with a side salad.

Nutritional analysis per serving (¼ chowder): calories 530 • fat 35 g • protein 38 g • carbs 15 g • fiber 2 g

## BROCCOLI CHEDDAR SOUP

*Makes 4 servings*

*Prep time: 10 minutes*

*Cook time: 30 minutes*

Broccoli and other cruciferous vegetables may have a big role in supporting detoxification, balancing your hormones, and providing plenty of fiber for your microbiome[16]—but that doesn't mean they can't be scrumptious as well! I find adding them to a creamy, high-fat soup is a great way to enjoy them. This one always reminds me of a restaurant-quality cream soup, but when I make it at home, I can use the highest-quality pastured dairy products to boost my nutrition and nutritional ketosis that much more. And I'll be honest, it is *so* easy to make, I imagine you'll find yourself preparing it weekly!

3 tablespoons butter or ghee

¼ cup diced yellow onion

2 cloves garlic, minced

4 cups broccoli, florets and tender parts of the stalk, peeled

3 cups Mineral Broth (page 197)

1 cup heavy cream

2 cups shredded cheddar cheese

¼ teaspoon sea salt

Pepper to taste

2 tablespoons full-fat Greek yogurt

### Toppings

Shredded cheddar cheese

Crumbled bacon

Chives, chopped

Add the butter to a heavy stockpot over medium heat. Add the onion and garlic and sauté for 2 to 3 minutes.

Add the broccoli and stir to coat with the fat.

Add the broth and bring it to a boil. Reduce the heat, simmer, and cover. Cook until the broccoli turns bright green and starts to become tender.

Use an immersion blender to puree the soup to your desired consistency, leaving some chunks of vegetable if you prefer.

With the heat very low, stir in the cream. Then begin adding the cheese ½ cup at a time, stirring until it is melted before adding the next batch. Once all the cheese has been mixed in and melted, remove from the heat. Taste and add more salt if necessary. Add pepper to taste.

Serve with Greek yogurt and your favorite keto toppings.

Nutritional analysis per serving: (¼ soup): calories 495 • fat 41 g • protein 23 g • carbs 9 g • fiber 2 g

## KETO CHILI

*Makes 4 servings*

*Prep time: 15 minutes*

*Cook time: 45 minutes*

Who doesn't love chili when it's also healthy for you at the same time, especially when you can top it with some Greek yogurt or sour cream for added fat, flavor, and probiotics? My advice: Break the rules on this recipe and make a double batch. Then freeze half for when you need a quick meal. Having my own "freezer meals" has helped me to stick with my keto lifestyle over the last few years— even when life gets busy. If I get home late, I always know I can have a nourishing keto meal ready for me and my family in a relatively short time. Final tip: If you can take the heat, add the cayenne pepper, which may promote vascular and metabolic health.[17]

3 tablespoons avocado oil

1 small onion, chopped

1 red bell pepper, chopped

1 zucchini, chopped

1 yellow squash, chopped

1 pound ground beef

¾ teaspoon salt

½ teaspoon pepper

2 teaspoons cumin

1 tablespoons chili powder

¼ teaspoon cayenne (optional)

5 cups spinach

One 10-ounce can diced tomatoes with green chilies

## Toppings

1 avocado, sliced

½ cup plain Greek yogurt

¾ cup fresh cilantro, chopped

4 tablespoons avocado oil (optional)

Heat a large sauté pan over medium heat and add the oil. Add the onion and cook for 5 minutes, until soft and translucent. Add the chopped pepper, zucchini, and squash and cook until they are soft and cooked through, stirring occasionally.

While the vegetables are cooking, brown the ground beef. Heat a Dutch oven or large pan over medium-high heat. Add the ground beef and start to brown it. Season with salt and pepper.

Add the cumin, chili powder, and cayenne, if desired, to the meat. Stir to combine.

When the meat is browned, add the spinach to the pan and cook until wilted, about 2 to 3 minutes.

Add the tomatoes and reduce the heat to medium-low; simmer for 10 minutes.

Add the vegetables to the ground beef and stir to combine. Serve topped with avocado, yogurt, parsley, and a drizzle of oil as desired. Serve with a side salad dressed in the remaining oil.

Nutritional analysis per serving (¼ chili): calories 655 • fat 57 g • protein 25 g • carbs 18 g • fiber 8 g

## CREAMY CURRIED CHICKEN SALAD WRAPS

*Makes 4 servings*

*Prep time: 15 minutes*

*Cook time: 3 minutes*

Chicken salad is one of my favorite ways to use up leftover chicken, and it's delicious when combined with Avocado Mayo and curry powder. In this recipe, I use a large collard leaf as a low-carb wrap and nutrient-dense alternative to a tortilla. If you've always found collard leaves to be bitter, you'll be blown away by how the fusion of other flavors, especially the onion and pickle, tones down that tang and makes it incredibly tasty instead!

¼ cup Avocado Mayo (page 200)

2 tablespoons tahini sauce (thin tahini with an equal amount water to create "sauce")

1 tablespoon curry powder

½ teaspoon sea salt

Pepper to taste

12 ounces cooked chicken thighs, skin on, diced

2 stalks celery, finely diced

¼ cup traditionally fermented pickles, finely diced

¼ cup red onion, finely diced (optional)

1 cup watercress, chopped

12 medium collard leaves

2 tablespoons Avocado Mayo (optional, for dipping) (page 200)

1 cup sauerkraut

Place the collard leaves with the thick-stem side up. Run a small knife parallel to the leaf, shaving off the thick part of the stem. Bring a large pot of water to a boil. Place the leaves into the boiling water. Let them cook for about 2 to 3 minutes (but no longer than that), remove, and set aside on a clean towel.

In a small mixing bowl, combine the Avocado Mayo, tahini sauce, curry powder, salt, and pepper. Stir to combine.

Place the diced chicken, celery, pickles, and onion in a large bowl. Add the mayo mixture to the chicken and mix to evenly coat the vegetables and chicken. Taste and season with more curry, salt, and pepper if you prefer more spice.

Take a cooled collard leaf and lay it on a flat surface. Scoop about ⅓ cup of chicken salad and place it in the center of the collard. Place a small handful of watercress over the chicken. Fold the wrap over the chicken mixture starting with the stem side, then fold the opposite toward the center, and then complete the other two sides as you would fold a wrap or a burrito.

Place three wraps on each plate and serve immediately with a side of sauerkraut. Dip the wraps in Avocado Mayo as desired.

Nutritional analysis per serving (3 wraps): calories 420 • fat 31 g • protein 22 g • carbs 13 g • fiber 1 g

# ROAST BEEF LETTUCE WRAPS

*Makes 4 servings*

*Prep time: 10 minutes*

Lettuce is such a great low-carb substitute for bread when making a sandwich, especially when you realize that bread usually brings less taste to a sandwich. What I love about romaine is both the crunch and how it makes it so easy to add additional greens to your plate. I think you'll discover the arugula nicely pairs with the roast beef because it is slightly bitter and peppery, but I urge you to play with your favorite condiments to really make this wrap your own!

1 pound sliced roast beef

8 slices bacon, cooked

1 avocado, sliced

4 cups mixed spring greens or arugula

4 tomatoes, sliced

¼ cup parsley, chopped

¼ cup basil, chopped

¼ teaspoon sea salt, divided

4 large romaine lettuce leaves

## Condiments

Mustard, Avocado Mayo (page 200), or tahini

1 cup sauerkraut

4 tablespoons olive oil (optional)

Divide the first 7 ingredients between each of the 4 lettuce leaves, add a sprinkle of sea salt, drizzle with up to 1 tablespoon of olive oil per wrap as desired, and roll up the leaves.

Enjoy with a side of sauerkraut.

Nutritional analysis per serving (1 wrap): calories 550 • fat 42 g • protein 32 g • carbs 12 g • fiber 4 g

# KETO GRILLED CHEESE

*Makes 4 servings*

*Prep time: 10 minutes*

*Cook time: 10 minutes*

What surprises many who have followed some form of ketogenic-based diet in the past is that you can absolutely continue to enjoy sandwiches on my program—especially if you make your own keto-friendly bread. My Keto Bread (page 224) makes this wonderful grilled cheese possible, but what really turns this classic lunch into a gourmet masterpiece is the addition of Gouda, avocado, and fresh basil. That combo makes it a sandwich worth paying for! Plus, the Gouda really brings both probiotics and plenty of good bacteria.[18]

¼ cup butter

8 slices Keto Bread (page 224)

¼ teaspoon smoked paprika

1 teaspoon sea salt

4 ounces Gouda, sliced

4 ounces cheddar cheese, sliced

1 avocado, thinly sliced

¼ cup chopped basil

⅓ cup broccoli sprouts

1 cup sauerkraut

3 tablespoons olive oil (optional)

Heat a pan over medium heat. Butter one side of each slice of bread. Sprinkle smoked paprika and salt on the buttered surfaces.

Place four slices of bread on the heated pan, buttered sides down. Lay the cheese slices, avocado, basil, and broccoli sprouts on the bread, dividing them evenly between the 4 slices. Top with the remaining 4 slices of bread, buttered sides up.

Slightly lower the heat and cook for a few minutes until golden brown; flip the sandwiches and repeat.

Serve with sauerkraut and a side salad. Drizzle with olive oil as desired.

Nutritional analysis per serving (1 sandwich): calories 600 • fat 53 g • protein 16 g • carbs 13 g • fiber 6 g

## KETO BREAD

*Makes one 8 x 4-inch loaf*

*Prep time: 10 minutes*

*Cook time: 30 minutes*

Bread—on keto? Yes, you heard correctly. Instead of relying on starchy, refined flour, my bread utilizes nutrient-dense almond flour as its base, which is higher in fat and protein than most other flours. Plus, the additional coconut flour boosts your fiber, while the eggs work like gluten to bind and help the bread rise. After exploring many versions of this bread, we finally found a winner that will wow you. Tip: For a less sweet version, try reducing the amount of monk fruit extract to suit your taste.

6 large eggs

¼ cup butter or ghee, melted

1 tablespoon whole-food MCT oil, plus extra for coating the pan

1½ cups almond flour

¼ cup coconut flour

3 teaspoons baking powder (aluminum-free)

½ teaspoon sea salt

1 teaspoon onion powder

1 teaspoon garlic powder

1 tablespoon monk fruit extract

Preheat oven to 375° F.

Separate the egg whites from the yolks. In a food processor blend the egg yolks, half of the egg whites, the melted butter, and the MCT oil until smooth. Pulse in the almond flour, coconut flour, baking powder, and salt until combined. The mixture will be thick.

Add the remaining egg whites and pulse until fully combined. Do not overmix or the bread texture will be tough.

Pour the dough into an oiled 8 x 4-inch loaf pan and bake for about 30 minutes. Test with a fork to see if the bread is cooked through. Cool on a wire rack for 5 to 10 minutes before removing from the pan and slicing.

Nutritional analysis per serving ($1/20$ of recipe): calories 113 • fat 9 g • protein 4 g • carbs 4g • fiber 2 g

# KETO BLT

*Makes 4 servings*

*Prep time: 10 minutes*

A traditional bacon, lettuce, and tomato sandwich is an American classic that everybody loves. But when you add in avocado, sprouts, and sauerkraut to elevate its taste and nutritional density even further, it goes from a staple to a sensation! This sandwich is sure to please, especially when you're in the mood for something dense, flavorful, and doughy!

8 pieces Keto Bread, toasting optional (page 224)

¼ cup Avocado Mayo (page 200)

½ cup broccoli sprouts

4 large lettuce leaves, torn into pieces

1 avocado

8 slices bacon, cooked

4 slices tomato

¼ teaspoon sea salt, divided

1 cup sauerkraut

Spread the Avocado Mayo on one side of each piece of Keto Bread.

Layer broccoli sprouts, lettuce, avocado, bacon, and tomato on 4 slices of the bread and top with the other piece of bread.

Add a sprinkle of sea salt to the avocado and tomato, if desired. Serve with a side of sauerkraut and a side salad.

Nutritional analysis per serving (1 sandwich): calories 460 • fat 40 g • protein 14 g • carbs • 17g • fiber 5 g

# KETO PB&J SANDWICH

*Makes 4 servings*

*Prep time: 10 minutes*

When I was growing up in Europe, PB&J sandwiches weren't a common thing. It wasn't until I became a mom that they entered my life. Now I enjoy them on occasion right alongside my kids— and this version is such a treat without any guilt attached, thanks to my sweet and tart Keto Raspberry Jam (page 226). My kids love this packed in their lunch for school except we swap out the peanut butter for sunbutter since our school is peanut free. But whether you have children or not, the kid in you will love this classic throwback!

8 slices Keto Bread, toasting optional (page 224)

½ cup natural peanut butter without added sugar

4 tablespoons Keto Raspberry Jam (page 226)

4 tablespoons whole-food MCT oil (optional)

Spread the peanut butter onto four slices of the Keto Bread and spread the Keto Raspberry Jam on the other four. Add the MCT oil as desired. Press the two slices of bread together to form a sandwich and enjoy.

Nutritional analysis per serving (1 sandwich): calories 420 • fat 41 g • protein 12 g • carbs 13 g • fiber 4 g

## KETO RASPBERRY JAM

*Makes 4 servings*

*Prep Time: 5 minutes*

*Cook Time: 10 minutes*

This jam is so simple and easy to make and doesn't contain a cup of sugar like most jam recipes. Instead, the flavor of the raspberries shines through. Try this in the Keto PB&J Sandwich (page 225), or place a dollop on the Key Lime Shortbread (page 272).

½ cup frozen raspberries

1 teaspoon lime juice

¼ teaspoon grated lime zest (optional)

Pinch of monk fruit extract (optional)

¼ teaspoon gelatin

Place a saucepan over medium heat. Add the raspberries, lime juice, lime zest, and monk fruit extract (if using). Cook until the mixture begins to simmer and the berries become soft, about 5 minutes.

Remove the berries from the heat and thoroughly mash with a fork. Alternatively, transfer to a blender to blend until smooth, using caution with the hot mixture and being sure to vent the blender; then return the mixture to the pan.

Warm the mixture over low heat and stir in the gelatin until all of the clumps have been broken up.

Remove the pan from the heat and let the jam cool. Then transfer it to a covered glass container and store it in the fridge for several hours until the jam sets. Store leftovers in the fridge.

Nutritional analysis per serving (1 tablespoon jam): calories 10 • fat 0 g • protein 0 g • carbs 2 g • fiber 0 g

## AVOCADO TOAST

*Makes 4 servings*

*Prep time: 15 minutes*

*Cook time: 5 minutes*

If I were to rank nature's most perfect foods, avocado would be at the top of my list! It is a great source of monounsaturated fat, similar to olive oil, and since it's a whole fruit, it also contains fiber.[19] For that reason, among others, avocado toast is hot right now and becoming a staple in many restaurants across the country. A crusty toasted piece of bread with creamy avocado is to die for, especially when topped with a runny egg and paired with a simple side salad.

4 slices Keto Bread (page 224)
¼ cup butter or ghee
4 eggs
2 avocados, sliced or mashed
½ teaspoon sea salt, divided
Pepper to taste
Red pepper flakes (optional)

8 cups spinach
2 cups shredded cabbage
2 tablespoons olive oil plus up to 4 additional tablespoons (optional)
Raw apple cider vinegar

Add 2 tablespoons of butter to a skillet over medium heat. Crack the eggs into the pan and cook to your liking.

While the eggs are cooking, toast four slices of Keto Bread, spreading each with ½ tablespoon butter.

Top each slice of bread with ½ a sliced or mashed avocado, 1 cooked egg, salt, pepper, red pepper flakes if using, and a drizzle of olive oil and vinegar. Serve with a side salad of the spinach and shredded cabbage dressed in olive oil and vinegar.

Nutritional analysis per serving (1 piece avocado toast): calories 680 • fat 67 g • protein 13 g • carbs 14 g • fiber 8 g

## KETO CRACKERS

*Makes 8 servings*

*Prep time: 15 minutes*

*Cook time: 30 minutes*

These crackers are so easy to make and so delicious that they have become a constant at my house as a snack for my kids and for myself. I often add these crackers to lunch when I want a little extra crunch and a hint more fiber to support my microbiome.

Tip: They are also amazing as an appetizer dipped in my Creamy Parsley Pesto (page 240).

| | |
|---|---|
| 1 egg | 2 teaspoons dried rosemary |
| ½ cup ground flaxseed | 1 teaspoon sea salt |
| 2 tablespoons chia seeds | Pinch of pepper |
| 1 teaspoon garlic powder | |

Preheat the oven to 300° F.

Whisk the egg in a mixing bowl. Add the other ingredients and mix until combined.

Place the dough between 2 pieces of parchment paper and use a rolling pin to roll the dough so that it is flat and even, about ⅛ of an inch thick.

Remove the top piece of parchment paper and use a knife to score the dough into 1½-inch squares.

Slide the parchment with the scored dough onto a baking sheet and bake for about 15 minutes.

Remove the baking sheet from the oven and break the crackers apart on the scored lines. Flip the crackers over and return them to the oven. Bake for another 10 to 12 minutes.

Let the crackers cool completely to harden.

Nutritional analysis per serving (⅛ batch of crackers): calories 70 • fat 5 g • protein 3 g • carbs 4 g • fiber 4 g

## MEATBALLS WITH ZUCCHINI NOODLES AND CLASSIC PESTO

*Makes 4 servings*

*Prep time: 30 minutes*

*Cook time: 25 minutes*

Full of antioxidant-rich herbs, this flavorful dish is a metabolic powerhouse. The Classic Pesto and Zucchini Noodles complement the Italian-style meatballs perfectly, and the wide variety of herbs helps reduce inflammation and supply just the right blend of earthy, fresh flavor to this to-die-for meal.

### Pork and Beef Meatballs

½ pound ground pork

½ pound ground beef

1 egg

1 tablespoon chopped parsley

1 clove garlic, minced

½ teaspoon dried thyme

½ teaspoon dried oregano

1 tablespoon tomato paste

½ teaspoon sea salt

¼ teaspoon pepper

Preheat the oven to 350° F.

Put all the ingredients into a large bowl and mix with your hands until well combined. Measure out about 2 tablespoons of the mixture and form into a ball; repeat with the remaining mixture. Place the balls on a parchment-lined baking sheet and bake until thoroughly cooked and browned on the top, about 20 to 25 minutes.

Serve with Classic Pesto (page 230) and Zucchini Noodles.

## Zucchini Noodles

2 large zucchini
1 tablespoon water

Cut the zucchini into long, thin "noodles" using a spiralizer, a julienne peeler, or a simple vegetable peeler.

Place the noodles and 1 tablespoon of water in a pan over low heat and cover. Gently steam until softened (about 5 minutes); then remove from heat and uncover.

## Classic Pesto

2 cups basil

2 tablespoons pine nuts

2 tablespoons Parmesan cheese (optional)

1 teaspoon lemon juice

1 teaspoon raw apple cider vinegar

¼ teaspoon sea salt

Pepper to taste

½ cup olive oil

1 cup sauerkraut

Place the basil, nuts, cheese if using, lemon juice, vinegar, salt, and pepper into a food processor and blend until well combined.

With the food processor still running, drizzle in the olive oil to make a creamy pesto. Taste and add more sea salt, if necessary.

Mix the pesto with the Zucchini Noodles and serve with the Pork and Beef Meatballs and a side of sauerkraut.

Nutritional analysis per serving (¼ pesto, noodles, and meatballs): calories 600 • fat 55 g • protein 26 g • carbs 8 g • fiber 2 g

## KETO BOLOGNESE

*Makes 4 servings*

*Prep time: 15 minutes*

*Cook time: 40 minutes*

I love that this warm and comforting Bolognese isn't just succulent, but is also so full of fiber-rich, carb-conservative vegetables that you stay in nutritional ketosis as well as being satisfied. It is such a versatile recipe and is easily one of my favorites. Fancy enough to serve to friends, yet rustic enough to be turned to in a pinch and enjoyed as a simple weeknight meal.

2 tablespoons butter or ghee

½ yellow onion, diced

2 celery stalks, finely chopped

1 zucchini, diced

1 yellow squash, diced

1 garlic clove, minced

1½ pounds ground beef

2 tablespoons tomato paste

1 cup tomatoes, diced

1 bell pepper (any color), diced

1 teaspoon sea salt

Pepper to taste

1 teaspoon dried oregano

¾ teaspoon red pepper flakes (optional)

2 cups parsley chopped

4 tablespoons olive oil (optional)

¼ cup Parmesan cheese (optional)

Heat the butter in a large skillet over high heat. Add the onion, celery, zucchini, squash, and garlic and stir to combine. Cook until softened (about 5 to 7 minutes). Lower the heat to low, stir in the beef, and cook for another 5 minutes.

Stir in the tomato paste, tomatoes, bell pepper, salt, pepper, oregano, and red pepper flakes if using. Cook another 25 minutes, adding in a little broth or water if the mixture starts getting thick. Tip: The flavor is enhanced the longer it simmers.

Serve over your favorite keto veggie, tossed with olive oil as desired: Zucchini Noodles (page 230), Cauliflower Rice (page 243), or sautéed spinach. Top with parsley and Parmesan cheese if desired.

Nutritional analysis per serving (¼ Keto Bolognese): calories 585 • fat 46 g • protein 29 g • carbs 12 g • fiber 4 g

## PEANUT SOUP WITH SHRIMP

*Makes 4 servings*

*Prep time: 15 minutes*

*Cook time: 30 minutes*

If you only have a few minutes to get dinner ready, this soup is for you. It's wonderfully simple, yet the flavors are so bold and undeniably delicious. The cinnamon, cumin, and turmeric actually work together to aid digestion while adding a nice punch of flavor that combines perfectly with the fresh ginger and garlic.

2 tablespoons avocado oil

½ white onion, chopped

3 cloves garlic

1 tablespoon grated fresh ginger

1 tablespoon coconut aminos

1 cup canned diced tomatoes

3 cups Easy Slow-Cooker Bone Broth (page 198)

½ cup salted natural peanut butter or sunbutter, no sugar added

½ teaspoon cinnamon

1 teaspoon cumin

¼ teaspoon turmeric

1 small head cauliflower, diced

2 cups cilantro, divided

1 pound shrimp, peeled and deveined

¼ teaspoon sea salt or more to taste

1 avocado, sliced

¼ cup sesame oil

¼ cup full-fat Greek yogurt (optional)

Heat the oil in a large stockpot over medium. Sauté the onion until translucent, about 5 minutes. Stir in the garlic and ginger.

Add the coconut aminos, tomatoes, broth, peanut butter, and spices and bring to a gentle simmer. Stir in the cauliflower and half of the cilantro; then cook at a gentle simmer for about 10 minutes.

Remove from the heat and carefully transfer the soup to a blender, working in batches if necessary. Vent the blender by removing the plug from the lid and covering the opening with a kitchen towel. Blend on medium until the soup is smooth.

Return the soup to the pot, add the shrimp, and cook over medium until opaque, about 3 minutes. Taste and add salt to taste. Divide the soup among four bowls and serve with sliced avocado, sesame oil, and yogurt if desired, with the remaining cilantro on top.

Nutritional analysis per serving (¼ soup): calories 610 • fat 49 g • protein 34 g • carbs 19 g • fiber 7 g

## COCONUT AND MACADAMIA NUT CHICKEN WITH ROASTED GREEN BEANS

*Makes 4 servings*

*Prep time: 10 minutes*

*Cook time: 45 minutes*

The macadamia nuts in this recipe are not just a rich source of anti-inflammatory polyphenols. They also may serve to prevent coronary artery disease (CAD),[20] and they help to give the chicken a buttery, crunchy texture that's both delectable and bistro-worthy. But what I most appreciate about this dish is the cilantro and lime toppings. It's quite honestly the perfect touch from a flavor perspective while also helping to protect your body from oxidative damage.

¾ cup macadamia nuts, finely ground in a food processor

¼ cup unsweetened shredded coconut

1 pound boneless, skin-on chicken breasts

¼ teaspoon sea salt

¼ teaspoon pepper

4 teaspoons Avocado Mayo (page 200)

Juice and grated zest of ½ lime

1 cup cilantro

1 cup sauerkraut

Preheat oven to 375° F.

Mix the macadamia nuts and coconut together in a small bowl and set aside. Place the chicken in a baking dish and sprinkle with salt and pepper. Spread each chicken breast with 1 teaspoon of Avocado Mayo.

Spread the macadamia-coconut mixture on the chicken.

Bake the chicken for 40 to 45 minutes on the center rack, being careful not to burn the macadamia nuts.

Serve with the fresh lime zest and juice. Top with cilantro. Serve with Roasted Green Beans and a side of sauerkraut.

### Roasted Green Beans

1 pound green beans, ends trimmed

1 tablespoon butter, melted

1 garlic clove, chopped

1 teaspoon fresh rosemary or thyme, chopped, or ½ teaspoon dried

¼ teaspoon salt

Preheat oven to 375° F.

Place the green beans in a bowl and toss with the butter, garlic, rosemary, and salt.

Spread the beans evenly on a baking sheet. Roast for about 15 to 20 minutes, until they are tender and just starting to turn brown.

Nutritional analysis per serving (1 breast with ¼ green beans): calories 630 • fat 52 g • protein 28 g • carbs 13 g • fiber 6 g

## GREENS PESTO CHICKEN

*Makes 4 servings*

*Prep time: 15 minutes*

*Cook time: 60 minutes*

Brussels sprouts have long been a favorite of mine because they are bursting with nutrients, with an especially high amount of both vitamins K and C. Plus they take on a taste that goes beyond delicious when served with chicken and pesto. To bring even more to your metabolic toolbox, I chose parsley as the base for this pesto to add additional antiaging flavonoids that lower your risk of cancer.[21]

1 pound brussels sprouts, halved

4 skin-on, bone-in chicken breasts

4 tablespoons olive oil

1 teaspoon dried thyme

Juice of ½ lemon

½ teaspoon sea salt

Pepper to taste

½ cup Greens Pesto (page 235)

Preheat oven to 350° F.

Place the brussels sprouts on a large baking sheet. Layer the chicken skin side up over the sprouts.

Drizzle the chicken and sprouts with oil and sprinkle them with the thyme, lemon juice, salt, and pepper. Cook for about an hour or until the juices run clear when you cut into the chicken, and the skin is golden.

Spread 2 tablespoon Greens Pesto on each chicken breast and serve over the roasted brussels sprouts.

**Greens Pesto**

½ bunch parsley

1 tablespoon fresh thyme

1 teaspoon fresh rosemary

2 garlic cloves, coarsely chopped

2 tablespoons whole-food MCT oil

3 tablespoons olive oil

Juice of ½ lemon

1 teaspoon raw apple cider vinegar

¼ teaspoon sea salt, plus more to taste

Combine all the ingredients in a food processor and blend until smooth.

Store leftovers in an airtight glass container in the refrigerator for up to 4 days.

Nutritional analysis per serving (¼ chicken with 2 tablespoons Greens Pesto and ¼ brussels sprouts): calories 580 • fat 47 g • protein 29 g • carbs 15 g • fiber 7 g

## GRILLED STEAK WITH MASHED "POTATOES"

*Makes 4 servings*

*Prep time: 15 minutes*

*Cook time: 15 minutes*

Steak and potatoes are the perfect comfort food for so many and fairly simple to throw together. This recipe turns that simplicity into something sensational by incorporating grass-fed steaks that are nutrient rich, especially in omega-3 fats that reduce inflammation and promote overall health. In fact, grass-fed beef has two to six times more omega-3 fatty acids than feed-lot beef![22] When served with creamy mashed cauliflower, this really is a decadent meal you can whip up any day of the week!

**For the Mashed "Potatoes"**

1 medium head cauliflower, cut into florets

2 tablespoons butter or ghee

¼ cup heavy cream

2 tablespoons full-fat Greek yogurt

½ cup shredded cheddar cheese

¼ teaspoon sea salt, or more to taste

Pepper to taste

2 tablespoons chopped parsley

2 tablespoons chopped chives

4 tablespoons olive oil (optional)

**For the Steak**

Four 4-ounce fatty steaks of choice, such as rib eye or New York strip

¼ teaspoon sea salt

Pepper to taste

4 teaspoons butter or ghee

Steam the cauliflower florets in a covered pot until fork-tender.

While the cauliflower is steaming, heat a grill or a grill pan over medium-high heat.

Sprinkle the steaks with salt and pepper on each side.

Place the steaks on the grill or grill pan and cook until golden brown, 4 to 5 minutes. Flip the steaks and cook for an additional 3 to 5 minutes (this time should yield a medium-rare steak), or until the desired degree of doneness.

Set steaks aside to rest.

While the steaks rest, transfer the cauliflower to a blender and add the butter, cream, yogurt, cheese, salt, and pepper. Blend until smooth. Alternatively, mash in the pan with a potato masher if you like a chunkier texture. Top with the parsley, chives, and a drizzle of olive oil as desired.

Serve each steak with a teaspoon of butter and extra sea salt.

Nutritional analysis per serving (1 steak and ¼ mashed "potato"): calories 570 • fat 48 g • protein 31 g • carbs 8 g • fiber 5 g

## PAN-FRIED ROSEMARY SALMON WITH SAUTÉED SPINACH

*Makes 4 servings*

*Prep time: 10 minutes*

*Cook time: 10 minutes*

As I mentioned before, I love salmon, which is why I try to incorporate it into my diet at least three times each week. But pulling that off means having a few great recipes on hand that are convenient and easy to clean up after. This homemade meal is exactly that: cooked simply with butter and herbs, it is super easy to prepare— and oh! Did I mention how tasty and good for you it is?

1 pound wild Alaskan salmon, cut into 4 fillets

¼ teaspoon sea salt

Pepper to taste

1 teaspoon fresh rosemary leaves, chopped

¼ cup butter or ghee, divided

8 cups spinach

1 avocado, quartered

1 cup sauerkraut

¼ cup olive oil (optional)

Sprinkle the salmon with salt and pepper.

Heat a large cast-iron or heavy-bottom skillet over medium-high heat. When hot, add half the butter and rosemary and stir to coat the bottom of the pan.

Add the salmon fillets skin side down and cook for about 4 minutes. Flip, add the remaining butter and spinach, cover the pan, and cook for another 4 minutes or until the salmon is opaque and cooked through and the spinach is wilted. Cooking times may vary depending on the thickness of the fish, so be careful not to overcook.

Serve with the butter and other liquid from the pan drizzled over the salmon and spinach. Top the fish with sliced avocado and a side of sauerkraut. Add olive oil for additional fat if desired.

Nutritional analysis per serving (1 salmon fillet and ¼ spinach): calories 510 • fat 42 g • protein 28 g • carbs 7 g • fiber 5 g

## GRASS-FED BURGER WITH JICAMA SLAW

*Makes 4 servings*

*Prep time: 15 minutes*

*Cook time: 15 minutes*

A good burger is so satisfying, and Jicama Slaw (page 239) really is the perfect accompaniment to boost your metabolism. That's because jicama contains inulin, one of the best prebiotic fibers you can feed healthy gut bacteria.[23] Plus it adds a cool and crisp contrast to the juicy, rich flavor of a grass-fed burger, making this a must-have meal you (and your microbiome) are sure to crave again and again.

1 pound ground beef

4 cloves garlic, minced

1 tablespoon dill, chopped

¼ teaspoon sea salt

1 tablespoon avocado oil

¼ cup Avocado Mayo (page 200)

4 collard leaves, blanched

8 slices tomato (optional)

1 cup sauerkraut

4 tablespoons olive oil

Mix the ground beef, garlic, dill, and salt in a bowl and then form into 4 patties.

Heat a heavy skillet over medium heat. Add the avocado oil to the skillet and cook burgers on both sides to preferred level of doneness.

Spread 1 tablespoon of Avocado Mayo on a collard leaf. Place a burger in the center of the leaf and 2 slices of tomato on top if desired. Wrap the collard around the burger. Repeat with the other 3 burgers and leaves and the remaining tomato. Serve with a side of Jicama Slaw and sauerkraut. Serve with olive oil for dipping, as desired.

### Jicama Slaw

⅛ small jicama (about 2 ounces), cut into matchsticks

1 cup shredded cabbage

1 tablespoon lime juice

¼ teaspoon sea salt

Pepper to taste

1 tablespoon Avocado Mayo (page 200)

2 tablespoons full-fat Greek yogurt

1 green onion

1 tablespoon mint, chopped

Add all ingredients to a bowl and mix until combined.

Refrigerate about 30 minutes before serving.

Nutritional analysis per serving (1 burger with ¼ slaw): calories 670 • fat 58 g • protein 27 g • carbs 16 g • fiber 7 g

## TURKEY BACON BURGER WITH CREAMY PARSLEY PESTO

*Makes 4 servings*

*Prep time: 15 minutes*

*Cook time: 25 minutes*

For a spin on a traditional burger, this turkey version incorporates fresh herbs and a delicious parsley pesto that gives it an extra burst of flavor. Personally, I love topping my burger with some traditionally fermented pickles to add some extra zing that supports gut health. While most people think that turkey is the leaner meat, you'll be happy to know that dark-meat turkey is often *higher* in fat than a traditional beef patty. Not only will the alternative to the standard beef patty delight your taste buds, but turkey offers a variety of nutrition too—it's an excellent source of B vitamins, selenium, and zinc. If you're craving a twist on the same old beef burger, this recipe will do the trick.

Note: If you're craving the traditional beef patty, you can easily swap that in here as well—just try to opt for grass-fed beef.

8 slices bacon

12 ounces ground turkey

2 cloves garlic, minced

2 tablespoons basil, chopped

¼ teaspoon sea salt

1 cup Creamy Parsley Pesto

4 collard leaves, blanched

⅓ cup sliced traditionally fermented pickles

1 cup sauerkraut

Cook the bacon over medium heat until crispy and set aside. Reserve half the bacon fat.

Mix bacon fat, turkey, garlic, basil, and salt in a bowl and form into 4 patties.

Heat a heavy skillet over medium heat and cook the burgers on both sides until no pink remains in the center.

Spread ¼ cup Creamy Parsley Pesto on one collard leaf. Place the burger in the center of the leaf, layer on the pickles, and wrap the collard around the burger. Repeat with the other 3 burgers. Serve with a side of sauerkraut.

**Creamy Parsley Pesto**

1 cup parsley

1 cup packed spinach

One 10-ounce jar artichoke hearts, drained

1 to 2 cloves garlic

¼ cup olive oil (or 2 tablespoons olive oil and 2 tablespoons whole-food MCT oil)

Juice of ½ lemon

¼ teaspoon sea salt or more to taste

⅓ cup walnuts

Pepper to taste

Parmesan cheese to taste

Place all ingredients in a food processor and process until creamy and smooth.

Store in an airtight glass container in the refrigerator up to 4 days.

Nutritional analysis per serving (1 burger with ¼ cup Creamy Parsley Pesto): calories 640 • fat 51 g • protein 34 g • carbs 12 g • fiber 4 g

## SEARED SCALLOPS WITH CILANTRO MINT SAUCE

*Makes 4 servings*

*Prep time: 20 minutes*

*Cook time: 5 minutes*

Scallops are such an excellent source of magnesium, potassium, and especially $B_{12}$, which helps promote a healthy nervous system and protect against chronic pain.[24] But what I love best is how they are also so easy to make. When possible, I prefer to pair scallops with the fresh Cilantro Mint Sauce that complements their buttery flavor so naturally.

### Scallops

1 pound sea scallops (fresh is best)

¼ teaspoon sea salt, or more as needed

1 tablespoon avocado oil

4 servings Zucchini Noodles (page 230)

### Cilantro Mint Sauce

*\*Makes about 1 cup*

2 cups packed cilantro

30 large mint leaves (about 5 sprigs)

⅓ cup olive oil

1 tablespoon fresh lime juice

1 teaspoon raw apple cider vinegar

2 teaspoons coconut aminos

Dash cayenne (optional)

¼ cup hemp seeds

4 tablespoons olive oil (optional)

Put the scallops on a paper towel–lined plate and salt all sides. Pat dry with a paper towel. Put the scallops in the refrigerator for 15 minutes, remove, and pat dry again.

Meanwhile, make the sauce: Place the cilantro, mint, ⅓ cup olive oil, lime juice, vinegar, coconut aminos, and cayenne if using in a food processor and mix until smooth and all the ingredients are incorporated.

Heat the avocado oil over medium-high heat in a cast-iron or stainless steel skillet. The oil should be very hot and spatter when a drop of water is added. Place the scallops in the pan and sear for 1 to 2 minutes until a golden-brown crust develops. Carefully flip the scallops and brown the second side, 1 to 2 minutes. You want a golden crust on both sides and for the scallops to be cooked throughout, but not overcooked in the center.

Place the cooked scallops on a paper towel–lined plate to drain briefly.

Serve immediately over Zucchini Noodles (page 230), topped with the Cilantro Mint Sauce, hemp seeds, and a drizzle of olive oil as desired.

Nutritional analysis per serving (¼ scallops and 1 serving Zucchini Noodles): calories 510 • fat 45 g • protein 19 g • carbs 9 g • fiber 2 g

## CHICKEN CURRY WITH CAULIFLOWER RICE

*Makes 4 servings*

*Prep time: 15 minutes*

*Cook time: 15 minutes*

The warm and aromatic flavors in this dish are always a crowd pleaser, especially when they are balanced with just the right amounts of both fresh cilantro and spinach. I can't get enough of traditional Indian spices like curry, turmeric, and ginger, not only for their amazing flavors, but also for how they all fight inflammation![25]

1 pound chicken thighs, cut into 1-inch cubes

1 tablespoon curry powder

1½ teaspoons salt

½ teaspoon pepper

2 tablespoons olive oil

½ medium onion, chopped

One 14-ounce can full-fat coconut milk

One 2-inch piece of ginger, chopped

One 1-inch piece of turmeric, chopped

4 garlic cloves

5 ounces spinach

¼ cup full-fat Greek yogurt

¼ cup cilantro

4 tablespoons olive oil (optional)

Toss chicken with curry powder, salt, and pepper in a medium bowl.

Heat 2 tablespoons olive oil in a large skillet over medium-high heat. Add the onion and cook until soft and translucent, a few minutes.

Blend the coconut milk, ginger, turmeric, and garlic in a blender until smooth.

Add the chicken and the coconut-milk mixture to the skillet and cook, stirring occasionally, until the chicken is completely cooked and the sauce has thickened, about 10 minutes.

Fold in the spinach; mix until wilted.

Serve over Cauliflower Rice (page 243) with a spoonful of yogurt and chopped cilantro on top. Drizzle with additional olive oil, as desired.

### Cauliflower Rice

1 head cauliflower, cut into chunks

2 tablespoons olive oil

¼ teaspoon sea salt

Pepper to taste

Place the cauliflower in a food processor and pulse until it is broken down into rice-size pieces.

Heat the oil in a large skillet over medium heat and add the cauliflower. Cover and cook until heated through, about 3 to 5 minutes. Remove the lid and fluff with a fork; season with salt and pepper.

Nutritional analysis per serving (¼ curry with ¼ Cauliflower Rice): calories 570 • fat 44 g • protein 31 g • carbs 20 g • fiber 5 g

## KETO CHICKEN WINGS

*Makes 4 servings*

*Prep time: 20 minutes*

*Cook time: 45 minutes*

I'll be the first to admit that chicken wings are always a big hit in my house, which is why I so enjoy this keto-friendly version. Even though they may take a little longer to prepare than other meals, the end result is worth the wait because they are crispy, crunchy, and beyond satisfying. My advice: Serve them with fresh veggies and my creamy Blue Cheese Dip to really take them to the next level!

1 tablespoon plus ¼ cup avocado oil, divided

1 pound chicken wings

¼ teaspoon sea salt

⅛ teaspoon pepper

½ teaspoon garlic powder

¼ teaspoon paprika or cayenne

¼ cup keto-approved, no sugar added hot sauce

4 large carrots, halved

8 celery stalks, halved

Preheat oven to 400° F. Line a large baking sheet with aluminum foil and set a wire rack inside. Brush the rack with 1 tablespoon avocado oil.

Pat the wings dry with a paper towel. Sprinkle with salt and pepper.

Bake for 45 minutes, until crispy and golden brown. The internal temperature should be around 170° F.

Mix the rest of the avocado oil with the seasonings and hot sauce in a large bowl. Then toss the hot wings in the mixture.

Serve with carrot and celery sticks and Blue Cheese Dip.

### Blue Cheese Dip

¼ cup Avocado Mayo (page 200) or full-fat Greek yogurt

½ cup sour cream

½ cup blue cheese crumbles

3 teaspoons lemon juice

¼ teaspoon garlic powder

¼ teaspoon sea salt

¼ teaspoon black pepper

2 tablespoons heavy cream (optional)

Place all the ingredients in a bowl and mix to combine. Include the cream for a thinner dip. Store covered in the fridge and serve cold.

Nutritional analysis per serving (¼ wings with Blue Cheese Dip and veggies): calories 500 • fat 46 g • protein 25 g • carbs 11 g • fiber 3 g

## FISH AND FRESH SLAW TACOS

*Makes 4 servings*

*Prep time: 15 minutes*

*Cook time: 10 minutes*

Wild Alaskan cod isn't just an abundant source of healthy fats; it's also *the* perfect fish for tacos—hands down! It's sturdy (so it doesn't fall apart easily when you cook it), and its mildness is a perfect match with any flavor—especially the savory cilantro-lime slaw you'll soon enjoy.

1 pound wild Alaskan cod

¼ cup avocado oil, divided

½ teaspoon sea salt, divided

2 tablespoons Avocado Mayo plus more for topping (optional) (page 200)

½ small red cabbage, cored and finely shredded

1 broccoli stalk, peeled and shredded

2 green onions, finely sliced

2 avocados, cubed

¼ cup chopped cilantro

Juice of 1 lime

1 teaspoon raw apple cider vinegar

8 large butter lettuce leaves

¼ cup pumpkin seeds (also known as pepitas)

¼ cup salsa of choice, home-made or prepared (no sugar added)

Heat a grill or grill pan over medium heat. Add 2 tablespoons of oil. Spread 1 tablespoon of oil over the cod and sprinkle with ¼ teaspoon salt. Place the fish on the grill, cover, and cook until the cod is opaque and just begins to flake, about 5 to 8 minutes depending on the thickness of the fillets.

In a bowl, mix the Avocado Mayo, cabbage, shredded broccoli stalk, green onion, avocado, cilantro, lime juice, vinegar, remaining avocado oil, and remaining salt, adding more salt if desired.

Divide the fish between the 4 lettuce leaves; then top with the slaw, pepitas, and 1 tablespoon of salsa. Add a dollop or more of Avocado Mayo to each one. Serve alongside any leftover slaw.

Nutritional analysis per serving (2 tacos): calories 602 • fat 52 g • protein 24 g • carbs 18 g • fiber 8 g

## CHICKEN AND WAFFLES

*Makes 4 servings*

*Prep time: 25 minutes*

*Cook time: 45 minutes*

When I've shared this dinner with others, they always tell me it almost feels like too much of a treat to be healthy, but it is! And although it may seem complicated to make, nothing could be further from the truth, especially if you make everything in the right order. The way I do it that always works: Once the chicken is cooking, *then* make the waffles, and this comforting dinner can be on the table in less than an hour.

### Oven-Fried Chicken

½ cup almond meal

½ teaspoon dried oregano

½ teaspoon paprika

½ teaspoon garlic powder

½ teaspoon sea salt

Pepper to taste

4 medium chicken drumsticks, skin on

2 tablespoons softened butter or ghee

Preheat the oven to 400° F. Line a baking sheet with parchment.

Mix together the almond meal, oregano, paprika, garlic powder, salt, and pepper in a shallow baking dish.

Rub each chicken drumstick with a generous spoonful of butter.

Dredge each one in the almond-meal mixture and place on the prepared baking sheet.

Bake for 45 minutes or until the chicken is cooked through and the juices run clear. The internal temperature should be around 170° F, and the skin will be crispy.

### Waffles

½ cup almond flour

¼ cup ground flaxseed

½ teaspoon baking soda

¼ teaspoon baking powder

¾ teaspoon Ceylon cinnamon

¼ teaspoon sea salt

1 egg, room temperature

⅛ cup full-fat coconut milk

1 tablespoon coconut oil or butter, melted

Grated zest of ½ lemon

Preheat the waffle iron.

Stir together the almond flour, flaxseed, baking soda, baking powder, cinnamon, and salt in a medium bowl and set aside.

Put egg, coconut milk, oil, and lemon zest into a blender and blend just until mixed and frothy.

Pour the wet ingredients into the dry ingredients and stir until just combined.

When the waffle iron is hot, pour ¼ of the batter into the iron and cook until crisp. Repeat three times.

Serve with Oven-Fried Chicken.

Nutritional analysis per serving (1 waffle with 1 drumstick): calories 530 • fat 44 g • protein 34 g • carbs 9 g • fiber 5 g

## FLANK STEAK WITH CHIMICHURRI SAUCE AND BAKED SPAGHETTI SQUASH WITH PARSLEY

*Makes 4 servings*

*Prep time: 15 minutes*

*Cook time: 50 minutes*

If you've never had chimichurri sauce—or tried to make it on your own—you are in for such an incredible experience with this recipe! Made from fresh veggies and herbs, this South American sauce is one of the easiest—and tastiest—ways I know to really pack more flavonoids into your diet, which benefits metabolic health.[26] Not only that, it is so rich in flavor, and when spooned over seared flank steak, the sauce brings out even more of the meat's mouthwatering flavor.

½ cup parsley, chopped

2 tablespoons fresh oregano or 1 teaspoon dried oregano

1 cup cilantro, chopped

4 cloves garlic

Pinch red pepper flakes

2 tablespoons lemon juice

1 tablespoon raw apple cider vinegar

½ small red onion, chopped

½ cup plus 2 tablespoons olive oil

½ teaspoon sea salt, divided between steak and sauce

¼ teaspoon pepper or to taste, divided between steak and sauce

2 tablespoons avocado oil

1 pound flank steak

1 large zucchini, diced

Heat a heavy skillet over medium heat.

Make the chimichurri sauce: Place the parsley, oregano, cilantro, garlic, red pepper flakes, lemon juice, vinegar, onion, olive oil, ¼ teaspoon salt, and ⅛ teaspoon pepper in a food processor and blend until smooth.

Season the flank steak with the remaining salt and pepper. Add 1 tablespoon of avocado oil to the hot skillet and then place the steak in the pan. Sear on the first side for about 3 to 4 minutes or until nicely browned and then flip to sear the second side for another 3 to 4 minutes. The steak will be medium rare.

Remove the steak when it reaches the desired level of doneness and let it rest for 5 to 10 minutes before slicing across the grain.

While the steak rests, cook the zucchini in the same pan, adding a little water or the remaining tablespoon of oil to loosen up any brown bits left from the steak. Cook until softened, about 3 to 5 minutes.

Serve the Flank Steak with chimichurri sauce, zucchini, and Baked Spaghetti Squash with Parsley.

### Baked Spaghetti Squash with Parsley

Half 3-pound spaghetti squash, seeds removed

1 tablespoon olive oil plus up to 3 additional tablespoons (optional)

¼ cup water

¼ teaspoon sea salt

¼ cup chopped parsley

Preheat oven to 350° F.

Place the squash, cut side down, in a large baking dish and add ¼ cup water. Bake for 45 to 50 minutes or until tender.

Remove squash from oven. Turn cut side up and cool for 10 minutes. Scrape the inside of the squash with a fork to create spaghetti-like strands.

Toss the strands of squash with the oil, salt, and parsley.

Nutritional analysis per serving (4 ounces steak with ¼ sauce and ¼ squash): calories 570 • fat 48 g • protein 26 g • carbs 12 g • fiber 3 g

## LEMON COCONUT CHICKEN WITH ROASTED BROCCOLI

*Makes 4 servings*

*Prep time: 15 minutes*

*Cook time: 55 minutes*

On busy days, recipes as easy as this one are a real lifesaver. What I love is that I can literally throw everything needed right in a pan and let my oven do the work while I tackle my to-do list—stopping to stir occasionally of course! And in addition to being quick and easy, this beautifully flavored dish is superb and so savory that it has instantly become a staple in my kitchen.

1½ heads broccoli, cut into small florets

2 tablespoons avocado oil plus 2 tablespoons (optional)

1 teaspoon fresh thyme or ½ teaspoon dried thyme

¾ teaspoon sea salt, divided

1 pound chicken thighs, skin on (Four 4-ounce chicken thighs)

1 small onion, halved and sliced

One 14-ounce can full-fat coconut milk

Juice of ½ lemon

1 teaspoon raw apple cider vinegar

Grated zest of 1 lemon

Dash of pepper

Preheat the oven to 350° F.

In a large mixing bowl, toss the broccoli with 2 tablespoons of the oil, the thyme, and ¼ teaspoon salt. Set aside.

Place the chicken, onion, coconut milk, lemon juice, vinegar, zest, remaining salt, and pepper in a baking dish.

Bake for 25 minutes; then flip the chicken and spoon the coconut milk over it.

Add the broccoli and cook for another 25 to 30 minutes until the broccoli is tender and the chicken is cooked through. Stir occasionally to ensure the onions do not burn.

Drizzle with additional avocado oil, as desired.

Nutritional analysis per serving (1 chicken thigh with ¼ broccoli): calories 435 • fat 35 g • protein 21 g • carbs 9 g • fiber 2 g

## GROUND LAMB PATTIES OVER CAULIFLOWER RICE WITH TZATZIKI

*Makes 4 servings*

*Prep time: 20 minutes*

*Cook time: 10 minutes*

Lamb is such an underestimated meat. It's rich in iron, high-quality protein, and saturated fats, in addition to niacin, zinc, and selenium. Spice it up with some cumin and curry powder, which both fight inflammation,[27] splash on some creamy Tzatziki sauce, which adds a burst of herby, lemony flavor, and you're left with a meal that's more like a celebration!

## Ground Lamb Patties

1 pound ground lamb

2 teaspoons cumin

1 teaspoon curry powder

1 teaspoon salt

¼ teaspoon pepper

2 tablespoons avocado oil

In a medium bowl, mix all the ingredients except the oil until thoroughly combined. Use your hands, but be aware that the curry powder will turn them yellow temporarily.

Heat a large skillet over medium-high heat and add the oil.

Form the lamb mixture into 8 patties and cook them for 4 to 5 minutes. Flip them over and cook another 4 to 5 minutes for medium or to the desired level of doneness.

Serve over Cauliflower Rice (page 243) with Tzatziki on top.

## Tzatziki

1 cup full-fat Greek yogurt

¼ cup olive oil

One 4-inch piece English cucumber, grated

1 tablespoon raw apple cider vinegar

1 tablespoon chopped dill

1 tablespoon chopped parsley

Grated zest of ½ lemon

1 tablespoon lemon juice

1 garlic clove, chopped

½ teaspoon salt

¼ teaspoon pepper

Place all the ingredients in a bowl and mix thoroughly with a fork to combine.

Nutritional analysis per serving (2 patties, ¼ Cauliflower Rice, and a generous ¼ cup Tzatziki): calories 520 • fat 46 g • protein 31 g • carbs 10 g • fiber 3 g

## ARUGULA SALAD WITH SOUTHWEST CHICKEN STRIPS AND SAUTÉED ZUCCHINI

*Makes 4 servings*

*Prep time: 20 minutes*

*Cook time: 35 minutes*

Salads are always a part on my dinner rotation because they're so versatile and easy to make. This Southwest version is no exception. It is flavorful and comes together so quickly (despite what may seem like a long list of ingredients) that I often find myself making it as a go-to meal.

Tip: Do not deny yourself adding avocado or a little Greek yogurt as a garnish for a splash of creaminess and healthy fat. If you need a little more healthy fat for fuel, drizzle a little extra olive oil over your salad at the very end.

2 tablespoons avocado oil

6 cups diced zucchini

2 teaspoons sea salt, divided

1 cup shredded, unsweetened coconut

2 tablespoons chili powder

½ teaspoon turmeric

Pinch cayenne

1 pound skin-on, boneless chicken thighs, cut into 1-inch strips

6 cups arugula

¼ cup chopped red onion

¼ cup olive oil plus additional 2 tablespoons (optional)

Juice of 1 lime

Sea salt to taste

Pepper to taste

Cilantro, chopped

1 avocado, cubed or ½ cup full-fat Greek yogurt

Preheat oven to 350° F.

Heat the avocado oil in a skillet over medium heat. Sauté the zucchini until fork-tender, about 3 to 5 minutes. Season with 1 teaspoon salt, toss to coat, and remove from heat.

Place the coconut, chili powder, remaining teaspoon of salt, turmeric, and cayenne in a food processor and pulse until the coconut looks like pebbles. Transfer the coconut mixture to a large plate.

Dredge the chicken strips in the coconut mixture and place them on a parchment-lined baking sheet. Bake the chicken for 25 to 30 minutes or until cooked through and at the desired level of crispiness for the skin.

Prepare the salad: Place the arugula, sautéed zucchini, and red onion in a large mixing bowl. Drizzle ¼ cup olive oil and lime juice over the salad and toss to combine. Season with salt and pepper. Divide the salad among four plates and place the chicken on top. Then garnish with cilantro and avocado or yogurt and the remaining olive oil if using.

Nutritional analysis per serving (¼ salad): calories 590 • fat 54 g • protein 27 g • carbs 16 g • fiber 6 g

## BEEF AND MUSHROOM MEATBALLS OVER SAUTÉED CABBAGE WITH MUSHROOM CREAM SAUCE

*Makes 4 servings*

*Prep time: 25 minutes*

*Cook time: 35 minutes*

This meal is truly warm and inviting, and it almost feels decadent because of its rich cream sauce. But don't let all that deliciousness deceive you, because the mushroom sauce is also rich in fiber and B vitamins that boost energy. And mushrooms are one of the few foods that contain vitamin D, which is essential for immune function.[28] The sauce perfectly complements the meatballs and cabbage, which is a fiber feast teeming with beneficial bacteria. If you need more fat for fuel, please add the additional ghee to make an extraordinarily indulgent sauce.

### Beef and Mushroom Meatballs

2 tablespoons coconut oil or avocado oil

1 onion, finely chopped

1 celery stalk, finely chopped

½ cup mushrooms, finely chopped

¼ cup chopped parsley

½ teaspoon white pepper

¾ teaspoon salt

1 tablespoon coconut aminos

1 egg, beaten

¼ cup shredded Parmesan cheese

1 pound ground beef

Preheat the oven to 400° F.

Heat a large skillet over medium heat and add the oil. Add the onion and cook until translucent, about 5 minutes. Add the celery and mushrooms and cook for another 5 minutes, just until they soften.

Transfer the onion mixture to a large bowl. Add the parsley, pepper, salt, coconut aminos, egg, cheese, and ground beef. Mix well with your hands until all the ingredients are incorporated.

Form into 2-inch balls and place on a parchment-lined baking sheet. Bake 20 to 25 minutes, until browned and cooked all the way through. Serve over Sautéed Cabbage with Mushroom Cream Sauce.

### Mushroom Cream Sauce

2 tablespoons butter

2 tablespoons ghee (optional)

1 small shallot, finely chopped

1 teaspoon fresh thyme or ½ teaspoon dried thyme

14 ounces mushrooms, sliced

¼ cup dry white wine

1 cup heavy cream

¼ teaspoon salt, plus more to taste

¼ teaspoon pepper, plus more to taste

Heat a sauté pan over medium heat. Add the butter, ghee if using, and shallot and cook for a few minutes until they turn translucent and soft. Mix in the thyme.

Slightly increase the heat and add the mushrooms. Cook until they are soft and brown, stirring occasionally.

Remove from the heat to add the wine and then return the pan to cook off the alcohol. Cook until most of the liquid has evaporated.

Add the cream and bring to a simmer. Reduce the heat to low. Allow to simmer until the sauce has slightly thickened and add salt and pepper to taste.

### Sautéed Cabbage

2 tablespoons butter or olive oil

½ small onion, chopped

1 garlic clove, chopped

1 small head cabbage, cored and shredded

½ teaspoon sea salt

Dash of pepper

Heat a large sauté pan over medium-high heat. Add the butter and onion. Cook for about 5 minutes, until the onions are soft and translucent.

Add the garlic, cabbage, salt, and pepper and sauté for 10 to 15 minutes, stirring occasionally, until the cabbage is tender.

Nutritional analysis per serving (¼ meatballs, sauce, and cabbage): calories 685 • fat 58 g • protein 27 g • carbs 14 g • fiber 4 g

## CAULI MAC 'N' CHEESE WITH STEAMED GREEN BEANS

*Makes 4 servings*

*Prep time: 15 minutes*

*Cook time: 20 minutes*

Cauliflower is such a great addition to a ketogenic diet, mainly because of its high fiber content and low carbohydrates. It's also one of the best foods you can eat to lower your risk of many chronic and cardiovascular diseases.[29] But what I might enjoy most is how its mild flavor lends itself so well to so many different recipes, and how it often takes on the essence of what it is paired with. That's what I relish about this recipe. The superfood works wonderfully in this creamy childhood favorite, especially when you add bacon for an extra boost of fats and flavor. This recipe is always a big hit!

8 slices bacon

1½ pounds cauliflower florets

⅓ cup milk

⅓ cup heavy cream

2 ounces full-fat ricotta cheese

2 tablespoons ghee or avocado oil

4 ounces cheddar cheese, shredded, divided

1 teaspoon Dijon mustard

1 teaspoon turmeric

⅛ teaspoon white pepper

½ teaspoon sea salt, plus more to taste

1 cup sauerkraut

Heat a large skillet over medium-low heat. Cook the bacon on both sides, being careful not to overcook. Set aside on a paper towel or a paper bag to absorb the grease. Once cool, chop the bacon into ½-inch pieces.

If you are using frozen cauliflower, make sure the florets are thawed before continuing. In a large saucepan, heat the milk and heavy cream over medium heat until it simmers. Add the ricotta, oil, and half the cheddar.

After the cheese has melted, remove the saucepan from the heat and add the mustard, turmeric, pepper, and salt. Add the cauliflower, return the pan to the heat, and toss to coat.

Once the cauliflower is coated and warmed through, sprinkle the remaining cheddar over the top. Stir in the bacon and serve hot. Serve with Steamed Green Beans and a side of sauerkraut. Drizzle with additional olive oil as desired.

### Steamed Green Beans

1 pound green beans, ends trimmed

Olive oil to taste

3 tablespoons chopped dill

Lemon juice to taste

¼ teaspoon sea salt

Place a few inches of water in a large saucepan with a steamer basket. (The water level should be just below the level of the basket.) Add the beans and bring the water to a boil. Lower the heat to medium and cover.

Steam about 5 minutes, or until the beans are tender and bright green.

Toss with desired amount of oil, dill, lemon juice, and salt.

Nutritional analysis per serving (¼ mac 'n' cheese and green beans): calories 635 • fat 58 g • protein 18 g • carbs 20 g • fiber 8 g

# BEEF STROGANOFF OVER BROCCOLI "RICE"

*Makes 4 servings*

*Prep time: 15 minutes*

*Cook time: 45 minutes*

I consider this quite possibly the perfect rustic meal. With a rich, flavorful broth, the stroganoff is hearty and delicious, plus it combines wonderfully with the broccoli rice. It takes a little extra work— and requires you to have a little bone broth at the ready—but once you're done, you'll have created a meal that's as restaurant-ready as it is refreshing and rejuvenating.

1 pound beef chuck

½ teaspoon sea salt

Pepper to taste

1 tablespoon olive oil

1 tablespoon butter

1 small onion, chopped

2 cloves garlic, chopped

6 ounces mushrooms, sliced

1 teaspoon fresh thyme

½ teaspoon onion powder

2 cups Easy Slow-Cooker Bone Broth (page 198)

½ cup full-fat Greek yogurt

¼ cup heavy cream

½ cup chopped parsley

Cut the beef into long strips and season with salt and pepper.

Heat the oil in a Dutch oven or large, heavy saucepan over medium-high heat. Working in batches, add the beef, brown it, then remove the beef from the pan and set it aside.

Add butter to the same pan and sauté the onion for 5 minutes until soft and translucent. Add the garlic, mushrooms, thyme, and onion powder.

Add the beef back to the pot; then add the Easy Slow-Cooker Bone Broth.

Cover and cook until the beef is cooked through and fork-tender and the liquid has reduced by at least half.

Add the yogurt and heavy cream and mix well. Turn off the heat.

Serve with Broccoli "Rice" and garnish with the parsley.

## Broccoli "Rice"

| | |
|---|---|
| 1 head broccoli, cut into chunks | ¼ teaspoon sea salt |
| 2 tablespoons olive oil | Pepper to taste |

Place the broccoli in a food processor and pulse until it is broken down into rice-size pieces.

Heat the oil in a large skillet over medium heat; then add the broccoli. Cover and cook until heated through (about 3 to 5 minutes).

Remove lid and fluff with a fork; then season with salt and pepper.

Nutritional analysis per serving (¼ stroganoff and "broccoli rice"): calories 520 • fat 39 g • protein 31 g • carbs 11 g • fiber 3 g

## PARMESAN CHICKEN TENDERS WITH ROASTED BRUSSELS SPROUTS

*Makes 4 servings*

*Prep time: 20 minutes*

*Cook time: 45 minutes*

Chicken tenders are always a top pick in any crowd, and this version is pretty close to a conventional preparation. The chicken is so crunchy on the outside and tender on the inside, and it's even better when dipped in Avocado Mayo (page 200). Then when you add the brussels sprouts and sauerkraut to this dish, they take it to an entirely different level metabolically, making the meal rich in prebiotics, probiotics, and sulforaphane, a phytochemical that lowers your risk of inflammation, oxidation, cancer—and even wrinkles![30]

1 pound skinless, boneless chicken breasts (about 2 large breasts) cut into strips

2 tablespoons avocado oil, plus more for greasing the wire rack

1 pound brussels sprouts, quartered

½ teaspoon sea salt, divided

Pepper to taste

1 egg

¾ cup grated Parmesan cheese

½ cup almond flour

¼ teaspoon garlic powder

¼ teaspoon dried oregano

1 cup sauerkraut

¼ cup Avocado Mayo (page 200)

Preheat oven to 400° F. Line a large baking sheet with aluminum foil and set a wire rack inside. Brush the rack with avocado oil and set aside.

Place the brussels sprouts in a baking dish and toss with the avocado oil, ¼ teaspoon salt, and pepper. Bake for 40 to 45 minutes until crispy on the outside and tender in the middle.

While the brussels sprouts begin to roast, set up two large, shallow bowls. In the first, crack the egg and beat it with a fork. In the second, mix the Parmesan cheese, almond flour, remaining ¼ teaspoon salt, garlic, and oregano.

Dip each strip of chicken in the egg mixture and then in the cheese mixture and set on the wire rack.

Bake the chicken strips with the brussels sprouts for 12 to 15 minutes until crispy and cooked through.

Serve the chicken and sprouts with a side of sauerkraut. Top with Avocado Mayo or place a spoonful on the side.

Nutritional analysis per serving (¼ tenders and brussels sprouts): calories 480 • fat 31 g • protein 38 g • carbs 14 g • fiber 6 g

# METABOMBS

## PUMPKIN PECAN PIE FAT BOMBS

*Makes 4 servings*

*Prep time: 10 minutes*

*Cook time: 10 minutes*

Pecans are one of my favorite nuts because of their creamy, fatty flavor and texture. They work perfectly in this fat bomb, which bursts with Thanksgiving flavors. Pecans are also high in anti-oxidants, including vitamin E, and important minerals such as manganese, zinc, and copper, which help to reduce inflammation and support immunity.[31]

1 tablespoon ghee, melted

⅓ cup pecans

⅛ teaspoon sea salt

¼ cup pumpkin (not pumpkin-pie filling; canned is okay, choose a BPA-free can)

½ teaspoon pumpkin-pie spice

¼ teaspoon monk fruit extract

⅛ teaspoon real maple extract (optional)

1 teaspoon collagen powder

2 tablespoons coconut butter

1 teaspoon coconut oil

Ceylon Cinnamon (for dusting)

Preheat the oven to 200° F.

Place the pecans on a parchment-lined baking sheet. Drizzle the ghee over the nuts, sprinkle with salt, and toss to coat. Lightly toast the nuts, waiting until you smell a nutty aroma, about 5 to 10 minutes. Set aside to cool.

When the nuts are at room temperature, place ¼ cup with the remaining ingredients in a blender and process until a sandy texture is formed.

Line a mini-muffin pan with parchment paper liners. Fill the muffin cups with the pecan mixture. Sprinkle each muffin with the remaining pecans and a dusting of cinnamon. Store in the fridge.

*Note: A little chunkiness from the pecans is fine and adds a delightful crunch to the texture.

Nutritional analysis per serving (3 bombs): calories 180 • fat 17 g • protein 2 g • carbs 6 g • fiber 1 g

## SMOKED SALMON BASIL BOMBS

*Makes 4 servings*

*Prep time: 20 minutes*

*Set time: 1 to 2 hours*

One way to help support the body with the transition into nutritional ketosis is to reduce or eliminate sweet flavors, especially for those prone to sugar cravings or with elevated blood sugar. These savory fat bombs help do just that, working as a high-fat snack or appetizer that doesn't tempt your sweet tooth while helping to give you a profound metabolic boost!

3 ounces goat cheese, room temperature

2 teaspoons olive oil

1 tablespoon chopped basil

1 teaspoon chopped dill

¼ teaspoon sea salt

⅛ teaspoon lemon juice

2 ounces wild Alaskan cold-smoked salmon, torn or cut into small pieces

¼ teaspoon capers or 1 teaspoon chopped Kalamata olives (optional)

In a medium bowl, combine the goat cheese, oil, basil, dill, salt, and lemon juice with a fork. Add the salmon and capers if using; then mix to combine.

With a spoon, scoop about 1 to 1½ tablespoons and roll into a ball. Place on a parchment-lined plate or tray. Repeat until all the mixture is used. Then refrigerate until firm, about 1 to 2 hours.

Store in a covered container in the refrigerator for up to one week. Best enjoyed cold since fat bombs soften at room temperature.

Nutritional analysis per serving (1 bomb): calories 61 • fat 8 g • protein 7 g • carbs 1 g • fiber 0 g

## JALAPEÑO LIME FAT BOMBS

*Makes 4 servings*

*Prep time: 10 minutes*

Spicy, salty, and cheesy, I promise this savory fat bomb will keep you satisfied between meals. And the heat of the jalapeños is worth braving to benefit your health—they've been recently linked to protecting against cell damage, diabetes, many cardiovascular disorders—and even Alzheimer's.[32]

Tip: I like to make a big batch of fat bombs each weekend to prepare for the upcoming week, so I have a keto-friendly snack ready to go whenever I need one.

4 ounces goat cheese, room temperature

2 tablespoons butter, room temperature

½ garlic clove, minced

½ teaspoon coconut aminos

2 tablespoons shredded Parmesan cheese

2 tablespoons shredded cheddar cheese

¼ to ½ jalapeño, halved, seeded, and finely chopped*

2 slices cooked bacon, finely chopped

Grated zest of ½ lime

Mash together the goat cheese and butter with a fork or in a food processor until smooth.

Mix in the garlic, coconut aminos, cheeses, jalapeño, bacon, and lime zest.

Divide the mixture into 4 fat bombs, rolling to form balls. Store in the refrigerator.

*Wash hands with hot, soapy water immediately after handling jalapeño—the juice can sting!

Nutritional analysis per serving (1 bomb): calories 170 • fat 14 g • protein 8 g • carbs 2 g • fiber 0 g

## POM BOMBS

*Makes 4 servings*

*Prep time: 10 minutes*

*Set time: 1 to 2 hours*

For those who love tart treats, the pomegranate powder in this recipe is a fun ingredient to play with. But the reason why I'm especially thrilled to share this recipe with you is that pomegranates also contain ellagic acid, a polyphenol compound that has been well studied for antioxidant properties, which may help to prevent chronic disease and the signs of aging.[33] Enjoy! You can find pomegranate powder at specialty food stores or online.

¼ cup macadamia nuts

2 tablespoons pomegranate powder

2 tablespoons coconut oil, softened but not completely melted

1 tablespoon collagen powder

½ teaspoon lemon juice

⅛ teaspoon sea salt

1 tablespoon cacao nibs

Finely shredded coconut

Place the macadamia nuts in a food processor and grind into a flour.

Add the pomegranate powder, coconut oil, collagen, lemon juice, and salt and process until combined and a ball begins to form.

Transfer the mixture to a bowl and stir in the cacao nibs.

Using a spoon, scoop out 1 tablespoon of the mixture at a time and roll it into a ball. Then roll the ball in the coconut and place it on a parchment-lined plate or tray. Repeat until all the mixture is used. Refrigerate until set, about 1 to 2 hours.

Store in a covered container in the refrigerator for up to 1 week. Best enjoyed cold since fat bombs soften at room temperature.

Nutritional analysis per serving (1 bomb): calories 190 • fat 18 g • protein 1 g • carbs 7 g • fiber 1 g

## PB&J BOMBS

*Makes 4 servings*

*Prep time: 10 minutes*

*Set time: 1 to 2 hours*

Biting into this rich fat bomb, you get the flavor of peanut butter and jelly. It's like eating peanut butter off a spoon, only way more satisfying in my opinion because of what awaits inside. The strawberries are high in fiber and relatively low in carbohydrates compared with other fruits,[34] making them fit (in moderation) perfectly into my plan.

¼ cup dry-roasted, salted peanuts

1 tablespoon coconut oil

1 tablespoon whole-food MCT oil

3 tablespoons fresh strawberries (about 2 to 3 medium strawberries)

2 tablespoons crushed, freeze-dried strawberries, plus more for dusting

1 teaspoon collagen powder

½ teaspoon monk fruit extract

⅛ teaspoon sea salt

Combine all the ingredients in a high-speed blender or food processor and process on high until completely smooth.

Pour into a mini-muffin pan, using about 1 tablespoon per muffin cup. Sprinkle crushed, freeze-dried strawberries on the top. Refrigerate until firm, about 1 to 2 hours.

Store in a covered container in the refrigerator for up to 1 week. Best enjoyed cold since fat bombs soften at room temperature.

Nutritional analysis per serving (1 bomb): calories 190 • fat 16 g • protein 4 g • carbs 7 g • fiber 2 g

## CHOCOLATE CHAI TRUFFLES

*Makes 4 servings*

*Prep time: 10 minutes*

*Set time: 1 to 2 hours*

The avocado is a little-known secret ingredient for making smooth and creamy chocolate truffles. But what's not secret is how I like to add spices to my diet as much as possible, even in treats. The spices in this fat bomb—which include cinnamon, nutmeg, ginger, and cardamom—are reminiscent of chai tea and offer important anti-inflammatory and immune-boosting compounds.[35]

2 tablespoons pecan butter

⅓ avocado

2 tablespoons coconut butter

1 tablespoon raw cacao powder

¼ teaspoon Ceylon cinnamon, plus more for dusting

Pinch nutmeg, plus more for dusting

Pinch ginger

Pinch cardamom

⅛ teaspoon sea salt

½ teaspoon real vanilla extract

½ teaspoon monk fruit extract

Combine all the ingredients in a food processor or high-speed blender and process on high until completely smooth and the batter begins to form a ball. The batter will be somewhat sticky.

Using a spoon, scoop out 1 generous tablespoon, roll it into a ball, and then place it on a parchment-lined plate or tray. Repeat until all the mixture is used; then refrigerate until firm, about 1 to 2 hours.

Lightly dust each ball with cinnamon and nutmeg.

Store in a covered container in the refrigerator for up to 1 week. Best enjoyed cold since fat bombs soften at room temperature.

Nutritional analysis per serving (1 bomb): calories 120 • fat 11 g • protein 1 g • carbs 5 g • fiber 2 g

# CRAVERTAMERS

## MAPLE WALNUT ICE CREAM

*Makes 4 servings*

*Prep time: 40 minutes*

*Cook time: 7 minutes*

*Set time: 2 to 4 hours*

This maple walnut twist on my keto ice cream as seen on *The Dr. Oz Show* and showcased on my blog is simply delicious! Hint: Think of this ice cream as a creamy fat bomb—meaning a little goes a long way (unlike traditional sugary ice cream where you need a big serving to feel satisfied)!

**Candied Walnuts**

¼ cup chopped walnuts
½ tablespoon coconut oil

¼ teaspoon monk fruit extract

## Ice Cream

2 eggs

3 egg yolks

1 teaspoon real vanilla extract

½ teaspoon real maple extract (or sub additional vanilla extract)

1 teaspoon monk fruit extract

⅓ cup coconut oil

2 tablespoons whole-food MCT oil

Make the candied walnuts: Combine the walnuts, coconut oil, and monk fruit extract in a saucepan.

Cook over medium heat 5 to 7 minutes, until the mixture starts to become light brown in color. Remove from heat and allow to cool, stirring frequently.

While the walnuts are cooling, make the ice cream: Combine the eggs, egg yolks, vanilla extract, maple extract, and monk fruit extract in a blender and blend until well combined.

Heat the coconut and MCT oil in a saucepan over medium heat until melted (or heat in the microwave for 45 seconds). With the blender on low, slowly add the hot oil to the egg mixture. Turn up to high and blend for 5 minutes.

Pour the ice cream mixture into a glass dish and place it in the freezer. After 30 to 45 minutes, when the ice cream is beginning to set, mix in the candied walnuts. Return to the freezer until firm, another 2 to 4 hours.*

To serve, let sit at room temperature for 10 minutes before scooping.

Note: Start with a half serving and work up as your body comes to tolerate MCT oil.

*Alternate method: After mixing the ingredients in the blender, transfer to an ice cream maker and process according to manufacturer instructions. Serve immediately.

Nutritional analysis per serving (¼ ice cream): calories 360 • fat 37 g • protein 6 g • carbs 2 g • fiber 1 g

## PEANUT BUTTER FROZEN YOGURT

*Makes 4 servings*

*Prep time: 15 minutes*

*Cook time: 5 minutes*

When a craving for a sweet treat strikes—and it will—this creamy treat never fails to hit the spot. The Greek yogurt and peanut butter provide a blend of protein and fat that keep your blood sugar stable, plus they give this dessert a wonderfully creamy texture that feels rich and tastes delish. By the way, the reason I prefer natural over conventional peanut butter is that it contains more of the plant compound resveratrol,[1] which may lower blood pressure and inflammation, protect against oxidative stress, and increase insulin sensitivity.

¼ cup heavy cream

½ tablespoon monk fruit extract

1⅓ cups full-fat Greek yogurt

¼ cup natural peanut butter without added sugar

¾ tablespoon whole-food MCT oil

Heat the heavy cream and monk fruit extract in a small pan.

Combine the yogurt, peanut butter, and MCT oil in a medium bowl, mixing until smooth.

Slowly add the warm cream to the peanut butter mixture and mix again until smooth.

Process in an ice cream maker according to the manufacturer's instructions.

Nutritional analysis per serving (a generous ½ cup): calories 240 • fat 20 g • protein 10 g • carbs 7 g • fiber 1 g

# DECADENT CHOCOLATE PUDDING WITH RASPBERRIES

*Makes 4 servings*

*Prep time: 10 minutes*

*Cook time: 5 minutes*

*Set time: 2 hours*

Perfect when you need a luxurious dessert, this chocolate pudding is sinfully indulgent and hands down one of my favorite desserts for a special occasion. The raw cacao not only gives this dessert its rich flavor, it also supplies important minerals and antioxidants that reduce stress and boost your immunity.[2]

Half 14-ounce can full-fat coconut milk (or sub ½ cup heavy cream)

1 cup unsweetened almond milk

¼ cup plus 2 tablespoons raw cacao powder

1 egg yolk

1 avocado

⅛ teaspoon sea salt

2 teaspoons monk fruit extract

1 teaspoon real vanilla extract

1 cup raspberries

Mint, for garnish

Combine the coconut milk, almond milk, cacao, egg yolk, avocado, salt, and monk fruit extract in a blender and blend until smooth.

Pour the mixture into a saucepan and cook over medium-low heat, whisking frequently, until the mixture begins to thicken so that it coats the back of a spoon. This should take about 5 minutes.*

Remove the pan from the heat, whisk in the vanilla extract, and pour the mixture into a glass dish. Refrigerate until set, at least 2 hours.

Serve topped with raspberries and mint.

*Note: Be sure not to let the mixture boil. If it starts to bubble, immediately remove it from the heat.

Nutritional analysis per serving (generous ⅓ cup): calories 210 • fat 20 g • protein 3 g • carbs 12 g • fiber 5 g

# SIMPLE BERRIES AND CREAM

*Makes 4 servings*

*Prep time: 5 minutes*

If you have very little time to throw something together for dessert, then this is the one for you. It only takes a few minutes and just five ingredients to enjoy this deliciously light treat. Simply keep a can of coconut milk in the fridge so that you're always ready to go! The berries supply fiber and reduce inflammation,[3] and I also find them to be a wonderful fruit to incorporate on days when you want an uncomplicated touch of sweetness to finish off your meal.

One 14-ounce can full-fat coconut milk, refrigerated overnight

1 teaspoon monk fruit extract (optional)

1 teaspoon real vanilla extract

1 cup fresh raspberries

1 cup fresh blackberries

Refrigerate the can of coconut milk overnight.

When ready to use, open the can and pour out the liquid (reserve for smoothies or another use). Scoop the hardened coconut cream into a mixing bowl and add the monk fruit extract and vanilla extract.

Combine using a stand mixer or hand mixer, slowly increasing the speed until it is at the highest. Mix 1 to 3 minutes.

Wash the berries and divide them between four bowls. Top with the whipped cream.

Nutritional analysis per serving (generous ¼ berries and cream): calories 250 • fat 20 g • protein 3 g • carbs 16 g • fiber 2 g

## KEY LIME SHORTBREAD

*Makes 12 servings*

*Prep time: 1 hour and 10 minutes*

*Cook time: 12 minutes*

There's just something so satisfying about a crunchy cookie. This shortbread won't disappoint you when it comes to crispness, and it has just the right amount of citrusy lime with a touch of sweetness. Bright and delicious, one cookie is perfect to satisfy your sweet tooth while maintaining nutritional ketosis. And why lime? Given the fruit's antibacterial, anticancer, antidiabetic, anti-inflammation, and antioxidant properties[4] that protect not just your heart, but your entire body from head to toe, the answer is as obvious as this shortbread is delicious!

¼ cup butter

¼ cup whole-food MCT oil

1 teaspoon lime juice

1 teaspoon grated lime zest

1 egg

2 teaspoons whole-leaf ground stevia or monk fruit extract

1½ cups almond flour

1 tablespoon coconut flour

¼ teaspoon salt

Cream butter, MCT oil, lime juice, lime zest, egg, and sweetener together using a mixer.

Add almond flour, coconut flour, and salt and mix well.

Roll the dough into a 2-inch diameter log, wrap it in parchment, and refrigerate it for 1 hour.

Preheat oven to 350° F.

Slice the log of dough into 12 round cookies (about ¼ inch thick) and place them on a parchment-lined cookie sheet. Flatten and shape each cookie as needed since they won't spread when baked.

Bake the cookies until slightly golden, about 10 to 12 minutes. Let them cool completely before removing them from the pan.

Store in an airtight container for up to five days.

Nutritional analysis per serving (1 cookie): calories 160 • fat 15 g • protein 4 g • carbs 3 g • fiber 2 g

# BONUS CRAVERTAMER BOMB: KETO LEMON CREAM SQUARES

*Makes 4 servings*

*Prep time: 10 minutes*

*Set time: 3 hours*

This incredible recipe is one you won't find in the meal plan—so those on my research trial never had the opportunity to experience it—but I simply couldn't resist sharing it with you once I discovered it at the end of my journey. Not only is it an absolute treat, but the grass-fed gelatin is essentially collagen that's great for your joints, supports gut health, boosts brain power, strengthens your nails, and improves your skin.

4 tablespoons grass-fed gelatin

Grated zest of 2 medium lemons

1½ cups boiling water

1 cup heavy cream

Lemon juice from 2 medium lemons (approximately ⅓ to ½ cup juice)

2 teaspoons monk fruit extract

Put 1 cup of room-temperature water in a large bowl and sprinkle the gelatin over the water. Let sit for 1 minute to soften.

Add the lemon zest to the bowl.

Pour the boiling water over the mixture in the bowl and begin stirring. Continue stirring until the gelatin is completely dissolved, about 5 minutes.

Stir in the cream, lemon juice, and monk fruit extract.

Pour the mixture into a 9 x 13-inch baking dish and put it in the fridge to set for at least 3 hours. Slice into squares and serve. Store leftover dessert in a covered glass container in the fridge.

Nutritional analysis per serving (¼ dessert): calories 110 • fat 12 g • protein 3 g • carbs 1 g • fiber 0 g

# SUPER FIBER
# BONUS RECIPES

## Achieve *More* with Artichokes

Ready to take your High Fiber Keto plan up a notch? I've got you covered with these high-fiber recipes featuring prebiotic fibers from both artichokes and Jerusalem artichokes. I strongly encourage you to incorporate these recipes into your meal plan as frequently as you can tolerate in order to reap the microbiome benefits and accelerate metabolic healing. I suggest following the meal plan as it is written for week one, and then beginning to incorporate these recipes in week two in order to ramp up your fiber intake more slowly.

Before we jump into these delicious recipes, here is the lowdown on artichokes to get you started.

# ARTICHOKES 101

## How to Select an Artichoke

Look for green, tightly packed leaves as a sign of freshness. The artichoke should feel firm. When comparing artichokes, choose one that feels heavy and solid for its size. The artichoke will be mostly green, perhaps with some purple depending on the variety.

Avoid artichokes that are splayed open or are browning on the tips of the leaves.

## How to Trim an Artichoke

Gently wash the artichoke in cool water.

Using a sharp knife or serrated knife, slice off the top inch of the artichoke. Using kitchen scissors, trim the pointy tip of each leaf. Slice off the stem if you prefer your artichoke to stand up in the pot or on your plate. If you prefer to eat the stem, you can simply trim the end and peel the stem.

If cooking whole, you can stop there. If you are preparing a recipe where you cut the artichoke into halves or quarters prior to cooking, be sure to remove the "choke," which is the area of tiny white and purple leaves on top of a white hairy area in the center of the artichoke. A spoon works nicely to scrape out the choke. Once removed you will see the artichoke heart below.

To prevent the leaves from browning, submerge the artichoke in a bowl of cold water with a squeeze of lemon while you prepare the other artichokes.

## How to Prepare an Artichoke—Three Ways

**Steam:** Place trimmed, whole artichokes in a steamer basket above boiling water and steam for 30 to 45 minutes, depending on their size. The artichokes are done when you can easily pull off one of the bottom leaves or insert a knife into the center (heart). Add citrus peel, herbs, or spices to the steaming water to impart flavor if desired.

**Roast:** Trim the artichokes, cut them in half, and remove the chokes. Brush the artichokes on all sides with your fat of choice—butter, ghee, olive oil, and avocado oil work well. Place in a baking dish and add any herbs, garlic, or other seasoning you like. Roast at 400° to 425° F until tender and the leaves come off easily, about 30 to 45 minutes. Alternatively, cook in the same way on a covered grill.

**Braise:** Heat a deep skillet over medium heat, add fat to the pan, add the trimmed and halved artichokes, and cook until lightly browned, about 5 minutes. Add Easy Slow-Cooker Bone Broth (page 198) or Mineral Broth (page 197) so it fills half of the pan, cover, and turn down the heat to medium-low. Cook until tender, about 25 to 35 minutes. Add salt, pepper, and any other seasonings you like and serve with the reduced broth.

## How to Eat an Artichoke

Pull off the outer leaves, dip into butter or sauce, and scrape the meat off each leaf with your teeth. When you get to the center, remove the choke (if it hasn't been removed prior to cooking) to reveal the heart. Cut the heart, dip, and eat.

> **Jerusalem artichokes** (or sunchokes) aren't artichokes at all, but the root of a plant in the sunflower family. Like artichokes, they are high in prebiotic fiber and low in carbs. They can be finely chopped or grated and eaten raw or cooked like other vegetables in a sauté, soup, or stew.

# LAMB CHOPS WITH ARTICHOKE PUREE

*Makes 4 servings*

*Prep time: 20 minutes*

*Cook time: 20 minutes*

This recipe highlights the delectable artichoke in a puree that's a perfect complement to succulent and juicy lamb chops. Packed with prebiotic fiber, this meal is not only delicious, it also provides a boost to the health of your microbiome and metabolism. Don't be intimidated by preparing the artichokes. It is quite simple after you do it once.

### Artichoke Puree

Try this puree as an accompaniment to chicken, fish, steak, or seafood. It is versatile and a great way to add fiber and fat to a low-carb keto meal. I like to roast the ingredients for this while I have other parts of a meal in the oven, and to make double so that I have leftovers.

One 14-ounce jar large artichoke hearts, drained

⅓ cup cubed Jerusalem artichokes (or substitute more cauliflower)

1 cup small cauliflower florets

6 cloves garlic, coarsely chopped

2 tablespoons plus ½ cup olive oil, divided

1 teaspoon lemon juice

½ teaspoon sea salt plus more to taste

Preheat oven to 425° F.

Toss the artichoke hearts, Jerusalem artichokes, cauliflower, and garlic with 2 tablespoons olive oil and roast for 18 to 20 minutes or until the vegetables begin to slightly brown and the cauliflower and Jerusalem artichokes are fork-tender.

Transfer the vegetables to a food processor and add the remaining olive oil, lemon juice and salt. Puree until smooth. Add more salt as needed.

### Seared Lamb Chops

This is such a simple recipe, but fancy enough for a special occasion or company. Cooking time will vary based on the size of your chops. Cooking to medium-rare is recommended, but be sure to not overcook. Fun fact: Lamb is particularly high in zinc and iron, even compared with other red meats. Enjoy!

8 lamb loin or rib chops

1 tablespoon fresh thyme leaves

½ teaspoon sea salt (or more)

¼ teaspoon pepper

4 tablespoons butter or ghee, divided

Rub the lamb chops with the thyme, salt, and pepper.

Heat a large, heavy skillet over medium-high heat, add half the butter and melt it, then add the lamb chops. Cook for 6 minutes, and then flip to cook the second side for about the same time or until the internal temperature is about 145° F.

Remove the lamb and let it rest for 5 minutes. Add the remaining butter to the pan to melt.

Serve the lamb with the pan butter drizzled over it and the Artichoke Puree.

Nutritional analysis per serving (¼ puree and 2 lamb chops): calories 610 • fat 55 g • protein 26 g • carbs 9 g • fiber 2 g

## ARTICHOKE HUMMUS

*Makes 4 servings*

*Prep time: 10 minutes*

This recipe is my favorite keto twist on a classic hummus, using packaged artichoke hearts instead of chickpeas. I kept the same traditional flavors with the tahini, olive oil, and garlic and just love the deep flavor of the artichoke base. Try this dip with Keto Crackers (page 228) or dip the leaves of steamed artichokes into Artichoke Hummus for an extra fiber boost!

12 to 14 ounces artichoke hearts, drained and pressed to remove excess water

⅓ cup Jerusalem artichokes, chopped

2 tablespoons tahini

¼ cup olive oil plus 2 tablespoons, divided

1 clove garlic

¾ teaspoon sea salt or more to taste

¼ teaspoon pepper

½ teaspoon cumin

½ teaspoon turmeric

1 teaspoon grated lemon zest

1 tablespoon lemon juice

Parsley, finely chopped, for garnish

Place the artichoke hearts, Jerusalem artichokes, tahini, ¼ cup olive oil, garlic, salt, pepper, cumin, turmeric, lemon zest, and lemon juice in a food processor and process until smooth, scraping down with a spatula as needed. If the texture is too thick, add a little more olive oil to loosen it.

Transfer to a bowl, drizzle with 2 tablespoons olive oil, and garnish with parsley.

Nutritional analysis per serving (¼ hummus): calories 260 • fat 25 g • protein 3 g • carbs 8 g • fiber 3 g

## SAVORY ARTICHOKE PORRIDGE

*Makes 4 servings*

*Prep time: 5 minutes*

*Cook time: 10 to 15 minutes*

I'm so excited to share this recipe with you! When I was younger, I loved a big bowl of oats, but used to make them savory with veggies and often a runny egg instead of the sweet bowls that are so common. This version uses a combination of cauliflower and artichoke instead of a grain for the porridge base. I top it with savory egg and butter. It is High Fiber Keto comfort food at its best!

1 head cauliflower (about 3 cups)

2 tablespoons butter or ghee plus more for drizzle

Two 12-ounce packages frozen artichoke hearts

1 tablespoon finely chopped fresh rosemary

1½ cup Easy Slow-Cooker Bone Broth (page 198) or Mineral Broth (page 197)

1 cup coconut cream

½ teaspoon sea salt or more to taste

2 cups fresh spinach

4 to 8 eggs, poached or fried

2 tablespoons coconut aminos

Red pepper flakes (optional)

Roughly chop the cauliflower into 2-inch chunks. Process in a blender or food processor until cauliflower becomes the consistency of rice. Place in a bowl lined with a paper towel and set aside.

Melt the butter in a heavy skillet over medium-high heat. Place the cauliflower rice, artichoke hearts, rosemary, broth, cream, and salt in the skillet and bring to a full boil.

Reduce the heat, cover, and simmer for about 5 to 7 minutes or until the artichokes are cooked through.

Place the artichoke mixture in a food processer and process until slightly chunky or your desired porridge texture.

To serve, place ¼ of the spinach on the bottom of each bowl. Fill the bowls with porridge (the heat from the porridge will wilt the spinach).

Top each bowl with 1 to 2 eggs and a little more butter. Drizzle with coconut aminos, sprinkle with red pepper flakes if using, and serve.

Nutritional analysis per serving (¼ porridge with 1 poached egg): calories 510 • fat 41 g • protein 18 g • carbs 22 g • fiber 9 g

## BREAKFAST BAKE WITH ARTICHOKE PESTO

*Makes 4 servings*

*Prep time: 15 minutes*

*Cook time: 50 minutes*

This breakfast bake is perfect for Sunday brunch and leftovers throughout the week. With four children to get ready in the morning, I need something fast, easy, and High Fiber Keto. This recipe has me covered. I like to top it with a generous dollop of pesto and pair it with some fresh greens. I feel good knowing I'm getting my fiber and greens first thing in the day.

8 slices bacon

½ small yellow onion, chopped

4 cloves garlic, chopped

3 cups spinach or arugula, coarsely chopped

20 ounces artichoke hearts, drained, patted dry, and chopped

12 large pastured eggs

½ cup cream or full-fat coconut milk

½ cup grated Parmesan cheese

¼ teaspoon sea salt plus more to taste

¼ teaspoon pepper

Preheat the oven to 350° F.

Cook the bacon in a heavy skillet. Remove the bacon, let it cool, and then crumble.

Add the onion to the bacon fat in the same skillet and sauté for 3 to 4 minutes. Add the garlic, spinach, and artichoke hearts. Stir to coat with fat and sauté for 1 to 2 minutes. The vegetables won't be thoroughly cooked.

Whisk the eggs in a large bowl. Add the cream and cheese. Arrange the vegetable mixture in a greased 9 x 13-inch baking dish, pour the egg mixture over it, and top with the crumbled bacon. Bake for 45 to 50 minutes or until the eggs are cooked through in the center.

Allow to cool before slicing. Top with Artichoke Pesto.

Nutritional analysis per serving (¼ bake with ¼ cup Artichoke Pesto): calories 540 • fat 41 g • protein 33 g • carbs 12 g • fiber 3 g

**Artichoke Pesto**

*Makes 6 servings*

*Prep time: 10 minutes*

If you want to make a sauce creamy, add some pureed artichoke hearts. It's one of my favorite ways to pack in this prebiotic fiber. This pesto uses the classic flavors of basil, olive oil, and garlic alongside some high-fiber variations, including pumpkin seeds and Jerusalem artichoke.

2 cups basil

Half 14-ounce jar artichoke hearts, drained

¼ cup pumpkin seeds

½ cup plus 2 tablespoons olive oil

¼ cup grated Parmesan cheese (optional)

1 tablespoon lemon juice

1 teaspoon grated lemon zest

½ teaspoon sea salt

½ teaspoon pepper or more to taste

Place all the ingredients in a food processor or high-speed blender and process until well combined and creamy.

Nutritional analysis per serving (¼ cup pesto): calories 270 • fat 27 g • protein 4 g • carbs 3 g • fiber 1 g

## BAKED ARTICHOKE SPINACH DIP

*Makes 4 servings*

*Prep time: 10 minutes*

*Cook time: 25 minutes*

Who doesn't love cheesy, savory artichoke dip? This keto version celebrates the spinach used in the classic version and is sure to wow and satisfy your family and guests with the uncanny rich and flavorful tastes and textures from the upgraded keto ingredients! It makes the perfect centerpiece for a platter of Keto Crackers (page 228) and sliced raw vegetables. If you happen to have any leftovers, I suggest using them as a filling for mushrooms or bell peppers. Just stuff your favorite veggies, bake for about 15 minutes, and you'll have a hearty High Fiber Keto meal in short order!

20 ounces artichoke hearts, drained and pressed to remove excess water, divided

⅓ cup chopped Jerusalem artichokes

2 cloves garlic

4 ounces cream cheese

¼ cup sour cream

1 cup shredded white cheddar cheese

4 cups chopped spinach

1 teaspoon salt

¼ teaspoon pepper

¼ teaspoon nutmeg

¼ cup grated Parmesan cheese

Preheat the oven to 375° F.

In a food processor combine 14 ounces (or 1 package) of the artichoke hearts, the Jerusalem artichokes, garlic, cream cheese, sour cream, and cheddar cheese and process until smooth.

Chop the remaining artichoke hearts and add to a bowl along with the spinach, salt, pepper, nutmeg, and artichoke-cheddar mixture. Stir to combine.

Place the mixture in an oven-safe baking dish, top with the Parmesan cheese, and bake for 20 to 25 minutes or until golden brown on top. Serve warm.

Nutritional analysis per serving (¼ dip): calories 310 • fat 22 g • protein 14 g • carbs 14 g • fiber 3 g

## STEAMED ARTICHOKES WITH LEMON TARRAGON BUTTER

*Makes 4 servings*

*Prep time: 10 minutes*

*Cook time: 30 to 45 minutes*

Simple and classic steamed artichokes dipped in a butter sauce are simply divine. They make the perfect appetizer or side for any meal. If you want to save time steaming the artichokes, try using a pressure cooker to save half the cooking time or more. Play with the herbs in the dipping sauce, and if you haven't tried ghee before, it works perfectly here.

4 large globe artichokes

6 lemon slices

½ cup butter or ghee

1 tablespoon lemon juice

1 tablespoon chopped tarragon

Trim the artichokes by removing the stem and thick lower leaves. Cut off the top inch of the artichoke and the tips of the pointy leaves. Rub the cut edges with the lemon slices or place the artichokes in a bowl of lemon water to prevent them from browning.

Place the artichokes in a steamer basket above boiling water, cover, and cook for about 30 to 45 minutes, or until the artichokes are tender, the leaves can be easily removed, and the heart can be pierced with a fork.

While the artichokes are cooking, melt the butter and combine it with the lemon juice and tarragon. Serve as a dipping sauce with the steamed artichokes.

Nutritional analysis per serving (1 steamed artichoke): calories 350 • fat 30 g • protein 5 g • carbs 17 g • fiber 9 g

## BAKED STUFFED ARTICHOKES

*Makes 4 servings*

*Prep time: 15 minutes*

*Cook time: 45 to 60 minutes*

This is my keto version of the classic Italian stuffed artichoke. Instead of high-carb breadcrumbs, use Keto Bread (page 224), which imparts even more flavor and texture to the dish. It may sound complicated, but once you try artichokes this way, they will be a staple on your High Fiber Keto plan, I promise!

4 slices Keto Bread, toasted (page 224)

1 teaspoon dried oregano

1 teaspoon dried basil

2 tablespoons chopped parsley

4 cloves garlic, minced

½ teaspoon sea salt

¼ teaspoon pepper

1 teaspoon grated lemon zest

¼ cup grated Parmesan cheese or 2 tablespoons nutritional yeast

¼ cup avocado oil plus 2 tablespoons, divided

4 large globe artichokes

6 lemon slices

1 bay leaf

4 cups mixed greens

Avocado Mayo, for dipping (page 200)

Make the stuffing: Pulse the Keto Bread in a food processor to form breadcrumbs. Add the oregano, basil, parsley, garlic, salt, pepper, lemon zest, and cheese and pulse again. Pulse in ¼ cup avocado oil and set aside.

Clean and prepare the artichokes by washing in cool water, cutting off the stems, cutting off the top 1 inch, and trimming the leaves. Rub the artichokes with the lemon slices to prevent browning. Optional: Remove the choke from the whole artichoke by opening up the center and spooning it out. You can also remove the choke later after eating the leaves.

Preheat the oven to 375° F.

Stuff each artichoke with ¼ of the stuffing mixture by pulling open the center and putting some in the middle and then pulling out each leaf and putting stuffing behind it.

Place 1 inch of water in a large Dutch oven and then stand the artichokes up inside. Drizzle with the remaining avocado oil and place the bay leaf and lemon slices in the water.

Cover the Dutch oven and bake for 45 to 60 minutes or until the artichokes are thoroughly cooked and tender. Serve on a bed of greens drizzled with avocado oil, with Avocado Mayo for dipping.

Nutritional analysis per serving (1 artichoke): calories 580 • fat 54 g • protein 12 g • carbs 20 g • fiber 9 g

# CONVERSION CHARTS

The recipes in this book use the standard United States method for measuring liquid and dry or solid ingredients (teaspoons, tablespoons, and cups). The following charts are provided to help cooks outside the U.S. successfully use these recipes. All equivalents are approximate.

| Standard Cup | Fine Powder (e.g., flour) | Grain (e.g., rice) | Granular (e.g., sugar) | Liquid Solids (e.g., butter) | Liquid (e.g., milk) |
|---|---|---|---|---|---|
| 1 | 140 g | 150 g | 190 g | 200 g | 240 ml |
| ¾ | 105 g | 113 g | 143 g | 150 g | 180 ml |
| ⅔ | 93 g | 100 g | 125 g | 133 g | 160 ml |
| ½ | 70 g | 75 g | 95 g | 100 g | 120 ml |
| 3 | 47 g | 50 g | 63 g | 67 g | 80 ml |
| ¼ | 35 g | 38 g | 48 g | 50 g | 60 ml |
| ⅛ | 18 g | 19 g | 24 g | 25 g | 30 ml |

| Useful Equivalents for Liquid Ingredients by Volume | | | | | |
|---|---|---|---|---|---|
| ¼ tsp | | | | 1 ml | |
| ½ tsp | | | | 2 ml | |
| 1 tsp | | | | 5 ml | |
| 3 tsp | 1 tbsp | | ½ fl oz | 15 ml | |
| | 2 tbsp | ⅛ cup | 1 fl oz | 30 ml | |
| | 4 tbsp | ¼ cup | 2 fl oz | 60 ml | |
| | 5⅓ tbsp | ⅓ cup | 3 fl oz | 80 ml | |
| | 8 tbsp | ½ cup | 4 fl oz | 120 ml | |
| | 10⅔ tbsp | ⅔ cup | 5 fl oz | 160 ml | |
| | 12 tbsp | ¾ cup | 6 fl oz | 180 ml | |
| | 16 tbsp | 1 cup | 8 fl oz | 240 ml | |
| | 1 pt | 2 cups | 16 fl oz | 480 ml | |
| | 1 qt | 4 cups | 32 fl oz | 960 ml | |
| | | | 33 fl oz | 1000 ml | 1 l |

| Useful Equivalents for Dry Ingredients by Weight | | |
|---|---|---|
| (To convert ounces to grams, multiply the number of ounces by 30.) | | |
| 1 oz | ¹⁄₁₆ lb | 30 g |
| 4 oz | ¼ lb | 120 g |
| 8 oz | ½ lb | 240 g |
| 12 oz | ¾ lb | 360 g |
| 16 oz | 1 lb | 480 g |

| Useful Equivalents for Cooking/Oven Temperatures | | | |
|---|---|---|---|
| Process | Fahrenheit | Celsius | Gas Mark |
| Freeze Water | 32° F | 0° C | |
| Room Temperature | 68° F | 20° C | |
| Boil Water | 212° F | 100° C | |
| Bake | 325° F | 160° C | 3 |
| | 350° F | 180° C | 4 |
| | 375° F | 190° C | 5 |
| | 400° F | 200° C | 6 |
| | 425° F | 220° C | 7 |
| | 450° F | 230° C | 8 |
| Broil | | | Grill |

| Useful Equivalents for Length | | | | |
|---|---|---|---|---|
| (To convert inches to centimeters, multiply the number of inches by 2.5.) | | | | |
| 1 in | | | 2.5 cm | |
| 6 in | ½ ft | | 15 cm | |
| 12 in | 1 ft | | 30 cm | |
| 36 in | 3 ft | 1 yd | 90 cm | |
| 40 in | | | 100 cm | 1 m |

# RESOURCES

## BOOKS

- *Glow15: A Science-Based Plan to Lose Weight, Revitalize Your Skin, and Invigorate Your Life* by Naomi Whittel, www.Glow15book.com
- *Lifespan: Why We Age—and Why We Don't Have To* by David A. Sinclair, Ph.D., with Matthew D. LaPlante
- *Quench: Beat Fatigue, Drop Weight, and Heal Your Body through the New Science of Optimum Hydration* by Dana Cohen, www.drdanacohen.com/quench

## DOCUSERIES

- *The Keto Woman* — naomiwhittel.com/ketowoman
- *The Real Skinny on Fat* — therealskinnyonfat.com

## KETONE TESTING

- Keto-Mojo — Recommended ketone and glucose testing meter, keto-mojo.com
- KETONIX — Recommended breath ketone analyzer, www.ketonix.com
- Ketostix — Recommended for ketone urine testing, available at Amazon.com

## FOLLOW NAOMI ON SOCIAL MEDIA

- Facebook — www.facebook.com/NaomiWhittel
- Instagram — Naomi Whittel
- YouTube — www.youtube.com/user/naomiwhittel

## PRODUCTS

- OMI Skin Nutrition — www.ominutrition.com
- Simply GOODFATS — www.simplygoodfats.com
- SlimFast Keto — slimfast.com/product_cat/keto

## SLEEP

- Dr. Michael Breus — thesleepdoctor.com

## SUPPLEMENTS

- NaomiWhittel.com

## PROFESSIONALS

- Dr. Dana Cohen — www.drdanacohen.com
- Dr. Dominic D'Agostino — www.ketonutrition.org
- Dr. Felice Gersh — www.felicelgershmd.com
- Dr. Michael Hoaglin — www.mikehoaglinmd.com
- Dr. Erika Schwartz — blog.drerika.com
- Dr. Brittanie Volk — blog.virtahealth.com/author/brittanievolk
- Beth Zupec-Kania — www.bethzupeckania.com

## APPS AND TOOLS

- 8fit.com
- Calorie, Carb & Fat Counter
- www.carbmanager.com
- Getmymacros.com
- Keto.app

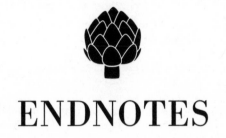

# ENDNOTES

## Introduction

1. M. Saklayen, "The Global Epidemic of the Metabolic Syndrome," *Current Hypertension Reports* 20, no. 2 (February 2018): 12, https://doi.org/10.1007/s11906-018-0812-z.

2. A. Ruiz, "Carbohydrate Intolerance," Merck Manual Professional Version (February 2018), https://www.merckmanuals.com/professional/gastrointestinal-disorders/malabsorption-syndromes/carbohydrate-intolerance.

## Chapter 1

1. G. Pizzino et al., "Oxidative Stress: Harms and Benefits for Human Health," *Oxidative Medicine and Cellular Longevity* 2017 (July 2017), https://doi.org/10.1155/2017/8416763.

2. N. Motamed et al., "Conicity Index and Waist-to-Hip Ratio Are Superior Obesity Indices in Predicting 10-Year Cardiovascular Risk Among Men and Women," *Clinical Cardiology* 38, no. 9, (September 2015): 527–34, https://doi.org/10.1002/clc.22437.

3. A. McPherron et al., "Increasing Muscle Mass to Improve Metabolism," *Adipocyte* 2, no. 2 (April 2013): 92–8, https://doi.org/10.4161/adip.22500.

4. Z. Aversa et al., "The Clinical Impact and Biological Mechanisms of Skeletal Muscle Aging," *Bone* 127, (October 2019): 26–36, https://doi.org/10.1016/j.bone.2019.05.021.

5. Z. Wang et al., "Specific Metabolic Rates of Major Organs and Tissues Across Adulthood: Evaluation by Mechanistic Model of Resting Energy Expenditure," *The American Journal of Clinical Nutrition* 92, no. 6 (December 2010): 1369–77, https://doi.org/10.3945/ajcn.2010.29885.

6.   J. Nicklas et al., "Association Between Changes in Postpartum Weight and Waist Circumference and Changes in Cardiometabolic Risk Factors among Women with Recent Gestational Diabetes," *Preventing Chronic Disease* 16, (April 2019): E47, https://doi.org/10.5888/pcd16.180308.

7.   Y. Ostchega et al., "Waist Circumference Measurement Methodology Study: National Health and Nutrition Examination Survey, 2016," *Vital Health Stat* 2, no. 182 (January 2019): 1–20, https://stacks.cdc.gov/view/cdc/61728.

8.   Y. Ostchega et al., "Waist Circumference Measurement Methodology Study: National Health and Nutrition Examination Survey, 2016," 1–20.

9.   E. Cespedes Feliciano et al., "Change in Dietary Patterns and Change in Waist Circumference and DXA Trunk Fat among Postmenopausal Women," *Obesity* 24, no. 10 (August 2016): 2176–84, https://doi.org/10.1002/oby.21589.

10.   R. Estruch et al., "Effect of a high-fat Mediterranean diet on bodyweight and waist circumference: a prespecified secondary outcomes analysis of the PREDIMED randomised controlled trial," *The Lancet Diabetes & Endocrinology* 7, no. 5 (May 2019): PE6-17, https://doi.org/10.1016/S2213-8587(19)30074-9.

11.   C. Emdin et al., "Genetic association of waist-to-hip ratio with cardiometabolic traits, type 2 diabetes and coronary heart disease," *The Journal of the American Medical Association* 317, no. 6 (February 2017): 626-34, https://doi.org/10.1001/jama.2016.21042.

12.   N. Motamed et al., "Conicity Index and Waist-to-Hip Ratio Are Superior Obesity Indices in Predicting 10-Year Cardiovascular Risk among Men and Women," 527–34, https://doi.org/10.1002/clc.22437.

13.   R. Mahmood, "Prediction of cardiovascular disease risk using framingham risk score among office workers, Iran, 2017," *Saudi J Kidney Dis Transpl* 29, no. 3 (May 2017): 608–14, https://doi.org/10.4103/1319-2442.235179.

14.   "Waist Circumference and Waist–Hip Ratio: Report of a WHO Expert Consultation" (Paper presented at World Health Organization, Geneva, December 2008).

15.   D. L. Waters, R. N. Baumgartner, P. J. Garry, and B. Vellas, "Advantages of Dietary, Exercise-Related, and Therapeutic Interventions to Prevent and Treat Sarcopenia in Adult Patients: An Update," *Clinical Interventions in Aging*, no. 5 (September 2010): 259–70.

16.   A. E. Locke et al. "Genetic Studies of Body Mass Index Yield New Insights for Obesity Biology," *Nature* 518 (February 2015): 197–206, https://doi.org/10.1038/nature14177.

17.   Z. Wang et al., "Specific Metabolic Rates of Major Organs and Tissues Across Adulthood: Evaluation by Mechanistic Model of Resting Energy Expenditure," 1369–77, https://doi.org/10.3945/ajcn.2010.29885.

18.   T. Greco et al., "Ketogenic diet decreases oxidative stress and improves mitochondrial respiratory complex activity," *Journal of Cerebral Blood Flow & Metabolism* 36, no. 9 (October 2015): 1603–13, https://doi.org/10.1177/0271678X15610584.

19.   S. F. Glotzbach and H. C. Heller, "Central nervous regulation of body temperature during sleep," *Science* 194, no. 4264 (October 1976): 537–39, https://doi.org/10.1126/science.973138.

20.   N. M. Punjabi et al., "Sleep-Disordered Breathing, Glucose Intolerance, and Insulin Resistance: The Sleep Heart Health Study," *American Journal of Epidemiology* 160, no. 6 (September 2004): 521–30, https://doi.org/10.1093/aje/kwh261.

21. N. Watson et al., "Recommended Amount of Sleep for a Healthy Adult: A Joint Consensus Statement of the American Academy of Sleep Medicine and Sleep Research Society," *Journal of Clinical Sleep Medicine* 11, no. 8 (June 2015): 931–52, http://dx.doi.org/10.5664/jcsm.4950.

22. M. Hert et al., "Metabolic syndrome in people with schizophrenia: a review," *World Psychiatry* 8, no. 1 (Feburary 2008): 15–22, https://www.ncbi.nlm.nih.gov/pubmed/19293950.

23. "Metabolic Syndrome," Metabolic Syndrome, Mayo Clinic, March 14, 2019, https://www.mayoclinic.org/diseases-conditions/metabolic-syndrome/diagnosis-treatment/drc-20351921.

24. Harriet Hall, "Inflammation: Both Friend and Foe," *Science-Based Medicine* (blog), December 27, 2011, https://sciencebasedmedicine.org/inflammation-both-friend-and-foe.

25. E. Kolaczkowska and P. Kubes, "Neutrophil Recruitment and Function in Health and Inflammation," *Nature Reviews Immunology* 13, no. 3 (March 2013): 159–75, https://doi.org/10.1038/nri3399.

26. I. Lalani, K. Bhol, and A. R. Ahmed, "Interleukin-10: Biology, Role in Inflammation and Autoimmunity," *Annals of Allergy, Asthma & Immunology* 79, no. 6 (December 1997): 469–84, https://doi.org/10.1016/S1081-1206(10)63052-9.

27. P. H. Wirtz and R. von Känel, "Psychological Stress, Inflammation, and Coronary Heart Disease," *Current Cardiology Reports* 19, no. 11 (September 2017): 111, https://doi.org/10.1007/s11886-017-0919-x.

28. F. L. Heppner, R. M. Ransohoff, and B. Becher, "Immune attack: the role of inflammation in Alzheimer disease," *Nature Reviews Neuroscience* 16, no. 6 (June 2015): 358–72, https://10.1038/nrn3880.

29. G. M. Slavich and M. R. Irwin, "From stress to inflammation and major depressive disorder: a social signal transduction theory of depression," *Psychological Bulletin* 140, no. 3 (May 2014): 774–815, https://doi.org/10.1037/a0035302.

30. Crusz and Balkwill, 584–96; Deng et al., 2016; Beatty et al., 2017.

31. G. M. Slavich, "Understanding inflammation, its regulation, and relevance for health: A top scientific and public priority," *Brain, Behavior, and Immunity* 45 (March 2015): 13–14, https://doi.org/10.1016/j.bbi.2014.10.012.

32. P. Sharma, "Inflammation and the Metabolic Syndrome," *Indian Journal of Clinical Biochemistry* 26, no. 4 (October 2011): 317–18, https://doi.org/10.1007/s12291-011-0175-6.

33. I. Aeberli et al., "Low to Moderate Sugar-Sweetened Beverage Consumption Impairs Glucose and Lipid Metabolism and Promotes Inflammation in Healthy Young Men: A Randomized Controlled Trial," *The American Journal of Clinical Nutrition* 94, no. 2 (August 2011): 479–85, https://doi.org/10.3945/ajcn.111.013540.

# Chapter 2

1. Office of Disease Prevention and Health Promotion, "Nutrition and Your Health: Dietary Guidelines for Americans," *Home and Garden Bulletin*, no. 232 (February 1980), https://health.gov/dietaryguidelines/1980thin.pdf?_ga=2.13475831.1718114262.1573498588-1282978834.1573498588.

2.  Jeff S. Volek and Stephen D. Phinney, *The Art and Science of Low Carbohydrate Living*, Lexington: Beyond Obesity, 2011.

3.  J. Volek, T. Noakes, and S. Phinney, "Rethinking fat as a fuel for endurance exercise," *European Journal of Sport Science* 15, no. 1 (October 2014): 13–20, https://doi.org/10.1080/17461391.2014.959564.

4.  J. DiNicolantonio, S. Lucan, and J. O'Keefe, "The Evidence for Saturated Fat and for Sugar Related to Coronary Heart Disease," *Progress in Cardiovascular Diseases* 58, no. 5 (March–April 2016): 464–72, https://doi.org/10.1016/j.pcad.2015.11.006.

5.  D. Mozaffarian, "Dietary and Policy Priorities for Cardiovascular Disease, Diabetes, and Obesity: A Comprehensive Review," *Circulation* 133, no. 2 (January 2016): 187–225, https://doi.org/10.1161/CIRCULATIONAHA.115.018585.

6.  F. M. Sacks et al., "Dietary Fats and Cardiovascular Disease: A Presidential Advisory from the American Heart Association," *Circulation* 136, no. 3 (July 2017): e1–e23, https://doi.org/10.1161/CIR.0000000000000510.

7.  C. W. Shih et al., "Changes in Blood Lipid Concentrations Associated with Changes in Intake of Dietary Saturated Fat in the Context of a Healthy Low-Carbohydrate Weight-Loss Diet: A Secondary Analysis of the Diet Intervention Examining the Factors Interacting with Treatment Success (DIETFITS) Trial," *The American Journal of Clinical Nutrition* 109, no. 2 (February 2019): 433–41, https://doi.org/10.1093/ajcn/nqy305.

8.  Brittanie M. Volk et al., "Effects of Step-Wise Increases in Dietary Carbohydrate on Circulating Saturated Fatty Acids and Palmitoleic Acid in Adults with Metabolic Syndrome," *PLoS ONE* 9, no. 11 (2014): e113605, https://doi.org/10.1371/journal.pone.0113605.

9.  Brittanie M. Volk et al., "Effects of Step-Wise Increases in Dietary Carbohydrate on Circulating Saturated Fatty Acids and Palmitoleic Acid in Adults with Metabolic Syndrome," *PLoS ONE* 9, no. 11 (2014): e113605, https://doi.org/10.1371/journal.pone.0113605.

10. Parker N. Hyde et al., "Dietary Carbohydrate Restriction Improves Metabolic Syndrome Independent of Weight Loss," *JCI Insight* 4, no. 12 (June 2019): e128308, https://doi.org/10.1172/jci.insight.128308.

11. J. C. Newman and E. Verdin, "ß-hydroxybutyrate: Much More than a Metabolite," *Diabetes Research and Clinical Practice* 106, no. 2 (November 2014): 173–181, https://doi.org/10.1016/j.diabres.2014.08.009.

12. B. Bailey, S. Phinney, and J. Volek, "The Science of Nutritional Ketosis and Appetite," *Virta Health* (blog), July 25, 2018, https://blog.virtahealth.com/ketosis-appetite-hunger.

13. D. S. Ludwig, "Dietary Fat: From Foe to Friend?" *Science*, 362, no. 6416 (November 2018): 764–70, https://doi.org/10.1126/science.aau2096.

14. Volek and Phinney, *The Art and Science of Low Carbohydrate Performance*.

15. K. H. Mikkelsen et al., "Systemic, Cerebral and Skeletal Muscle Ketone Body and Energy Metabolism During Acute Hyper-d-ß-Hydroxybutyratemia in Post-Absorptive Healthy Males," *The Journal of Clinical Endocrinology & Metabolism* 100, no. 2 (February 2015): 636–43, https://doi.org/10.1210/jc.2014-2608.

16. C. J. dC. Harvey, G. M. Schofield, M. Williden, "The Use of Nutritional Supplements to Induce Ketosis and Reduce Symptoms Associated with Keto-Induction: A Narrative Review," *PeerJ* 6 (March 2018): e4488, https://doi.org/10.7717/peerj.4488.

17. E. P. G. Vining et al., "A Multicenter Study of the Efficacy of the Ketogenic Diet," *Archives of Neurology* 55, no. 11 (November 1998): 1433–7, https://doi.org/10.1001/archneur.55.11.1433.

18. A. M. Sherman et al., "Dietary Adherence: Characteristics and Interventions," *Controlled Clinical Trials* 21, no. S5 (October 2000): S206–11, https://doi.org/10.1016/s0197-2456(00)00080-5.

19. B. M. Popkin, K. E. D'Anci, and I. H. Rosenberg, "Water, Hydration, and Health," *Nutrition Reviews* 68, no. 8 (August 2010): 439–58, https://doi.org/10.1111/j.1753-4887.2010.00304.x.

20. S. Kielb et al., "Nephrolithiasis associated with the ketogenic diet," *The Journal of Urology* 164, no. 2 (August 2000): 464–6, https://doi.org/10.1016/S0022-5347(05)67400-9.

21. B. S. Fuehrlein et al., "Differential Metabolic Effects of Saturated Versus Polyunsaturated Fats in Ketogenic Diets," *The Journal of Clinical Endocrinology & Metabolism* 89, no. 4 (April 2004): 1641–5, https://doi.org/10.1210/jc.2003-031796.

22. M. de Lorgeril and P. Salen, "New Insights into the Health Effects of Dietary Saturated and Omega-6 and Omega-3 Polyunsaturated Fatty Acids," *BMC Medicine* 10 (May 2012): 50, https://doi.org/10.1186/1741-7015-10-50.

23. M. Lagarde et al., "Oxygenation of Polyunsaturated Fatty Acids and Oxidative Stress within Blood Platelets," *Biochimica et Biophysica Acta (BBA): Molecular and Cell Biology of Lipids* 1863, no. 6 (June 2018): 651–6, https://doi.org/10.1016/j.bbalip.2018.03.005.

24. E. G. Neal, B. Zupec-Kania, and H. H. Pfeifer, "Carnitine, Nutritional Supplementation and Discontinuation of Ketogenic Diet Therapies," *Epilepsy Research* 100, no. 3 (July 2012): 267–71, https://doi.org/10.1016/j.eplepsyres.2012.04.021.

25. J. B. Calton, "Prevalence of Micronutrient Deficiency in Popular Diet Plans," *Journal of the International Society of Sports Nutrition* 7 (June 2010): 24, https://doi.org/10.1186/1550-2783-7-24.

# Chapter 3

1. S. McGuire, "Scientific Report of the 2015 Dietary Guidelines Advisory Committee, Washington, DC: US Departments of Agriculture and Health and Human Services, 2015," *Advances in Nutrition* 7, no. 1 (January 2016): 202–4, https://doi.org/10.3945/an.115.011684.

2. J. K. Schmier et al., "Cost Savings of Reduced Constipation Rates Attributed to Increased Dietary Fiber Intakes: A Decision-Analytic Model," *BMC Public Health* 14, no. 374 (April 2014), https://doi.org/10.1186/1471-2458-14-374.

3. D. Mandaliya, S. Patel, and S. Seshadri, "Fiber in Our Diet and Its Role in Health and Disease," in *Functional Food and Human Health*, ed. Vibha Rani and Umesh C. S. Yadav, Singapore: Springer, (2018): 247–55, https://doi.org/10.1007/978-981-13-1123-9.

4.  W. Dahl and M. Stewart, "Position of the Academy of Nutrition and Dietetics: Health Implications of Dietary Fiber," *Journal of the Academy of Nutrition and Dietetics* 115, no. 11 (November 2015): 1861–70, https://doi.org/10.1016/j.jand .2015.09.003.

5.  Kya N. Grooms et al., "Dietary Fiber Intake and Cardiometabolic Risks among US Adults, NHANES 1999–2010," *The American Journal of Medicine* 126, no. 12 (December 2013): 1059–67, https://doi.org/10.1016/j.amjmed.2013.07.023.

6.  A. Aleixandre and M. Miguel, "Dietary fiber and blood pressure control," *Food & Function* 7, no. 4 (April 2016): 1864–71, https://doi.org/10.1039/c5fo00950b.

7.  A. Reynolds et al., "Carbohydrate Quality and Human Health: A Series of Systematic Reviews and Meta-Analyses," *The Lancet* 393, no. 10170 (February 2019): 434–45, https://doi.org/10.1016/S0140-6736(18)31809-9.

8.  C. R. McGill, V. L. Fulgoni III, and L. Devareddy, "Ten-Year Trends in Fiber and Whole Grain Intakes and Food Sources for the United States Population: National Health and Nutrition Examination Survey 2001–2010," *Nutrients* 7, no. 2 (February 2015): 1119–30, https://doi.org/10.3390/nu7021119.

9.  Reynolds et al., "Carbohydrate Quality and Human Health: A Series of Systematic Reviews and Meta-Analyses," 434–45.

10. McGill, Fulgoni, and Devareddy, "Ten-Year Trends in Fiberand Whole Grain Intakes and Food Sources for the United States Population: National Health and Nutrition Examination Survey 2001–2010," 1119–30.

11. F. Calvaleri and E. Bashar, "Potential Synergies of ß-Hydroxybutyrate and Butyrate on the Modulation of Metabolism, Inflammation, Cognition, and General Health," *Journal of Nutrition and Metabolism* (April 2018) 7195760, https://doi.org/10.1155/2018/7195760.

12. H. Ohira, W. Tsutsui, and Y. Fujioka, "Are Short Chain Fatty Acids in Gut Microbiota Defensive Players for Inflammation and Atherosclerosis?," *Journal of Atherosclerosis and Thrombosis* 24, no. 7 (July 2017): 660–72, https://doi. org/10.5551/jat.RV17006.

13. Y. Zhang et al., "Butyrate promotes slow-twitch myofiber formation and mitochondrial biogenesis in finishing pigs via inducing specific microRNAs and PGC-1α expression," *Journal of Animal Science* 97, no. 8 (August 2019): 3180–92, https://doi.org/10.1093/jas/skz187.

14. M. Dave et al., "The Human Gut Microbiome: Current Knowledge, Challenges, and Future Directions," *Translational Research* 160, no. 4 (October 2012): 246–57, https://doi.org/10.1016/j.trsl.2012.05.003.

15. C. Palmer et al., "Development of the Human Infant Intestinal Microbiota," *PLoS Biol* 5, no. 7 (June 2007): e177, https://doi.org/10.1371/journal.pbio.0050177.

16. H. Fang, J. Kang, and D. Zhang, "Microbial Production of Vitamin B12: A Review and Future Perspectives," *Microbial Cell Factories* 16, no. 1 (January 2017): 15, https://doi.org/10.1186/s12934-017-0631-y.

17. R. K. Singh et al., "Influence of Diet on the Gut Microbiome and Implications for Human Health," *Journal of Translational Medicine* 15 (April 2017): 73, https:// doi.org/10.1186/s12967-017-1175-y.

18. A. B. Shreiner, J. Y. Kao, and V. B. Young, "The Gut Microbiome in Health and in Disease," *Current Opinion in Gastroenterology* 31, no. 1 (January 2015): 69–75, https://doi.org/10.1097/MOG.0000000000000139.

19. G. Vighi et al., "Allergy and the gastrointestinal system," *Clinical & Experimental Immunology* 153, no. s1 (September 2008): 3–6, https://doi.org/10.1111/j.1365 -2249.2008.03713.x.

20. S. Tuddenham and C. L. Sears, "The Intestinal Microbiome and Health," *Current Opinion in Infectious Diseases* 28, no. 5 (October 2015): 464–70, https://doi.org/ 10.1097/QCO.0000000000000196.

21. L. A. David et al., "Diet Rapidly and Reproducibly Alters the Human Gut Microbiome," *Nature* 505 (January 2014): 559–63, https://doi.org/10.1038/ nature12820.

22. J. Slavin, "Fiber and Prebiotics: Mechanisms and Health Benefits," *Nutrients* 5, no. 4 (April 2013): 1417–35, https://doi.org/10.3390/nu5041417.

23. L. Niittynen, K. Kajander, and R. Korpela, "Galacto-Oligosaccharides and Bowel Function," *Scandinavian Journal of Food & Nutrition* 51, no. 2 (June 2007): 62–6, https://doi.org/10.1080/17482970701414596.

24. D. Garrido et al., "Comparative Transcriptomics Reveals Key Differences in the Response to Milk Oligosaccharides of Infant Gut-Associated Bifidobacterial," *Scientific Reports* 5 (September 2015): 13517, https://doi.org/10.1038/srep13517.

25. Kelsey Marksteiner, "Do Polyphenols Improve Your Gut Bacteria?" *Chriskresser .com*, June 16, 2019, www.chriskresser.com/do-polyphenols-improve-your-gut -bacteria/.

26. N. Hayek, "Chocolate, Gut Microbiota, and Human Health," *Frontiers in Pharmacology* 4 (February 2013): 11, https://doi.org/10.3389/fphar.2013.00011.

# Chapter 4

1. A. Ruiz, "Carbohydrate Intolerance," *Merck Manual Professional Version,* revised February 2018: https://www.merckmanuals.com/professional/gastrointestinal-disorders/malabsorption-syndromes/carbohydrate-intolerance.

2. McGuire, *Advances in Nutrition,* 7: 202–204.

3. R. Sender, S. Fuchs, and R. Milo, "Revised Estimates for the Number of Human and Bacteria Cells in the Body," *PLoS Biology* 14, no. 8 (August 2016): e1002533, https://doi.org/10.1371/journal.pbio.1002533.

4. M. E. Raichle and D. A. Gusnard, "Appraising the Brain's Energy Budget," *Proceedings of the National Academy of Sciences of the United States of America* 99, no. 16 (August 2002): 10237–9, https://doi.org/10.1073/pnas.172399499.

5. S. D. Hewagalamulage et al., "Stress, Cortisol, and Obesity: A Role for Cortisol Responsiveness in Identifying Individuals Prone to Obesity," *Domestic Animal Endocrinology* 56, Supplement (July 2016): S112–20, https://doi.org/10.1016/ j.domaniend.2016.03.004.

6. A. Spivey, "Lose Sleep, Gain Weight: Another Piece of the Obesity Puzzle," *Environmental Health Perspectives* 118, no. 1 (January 2010): A28–A33, https:// doi.org/10.1289/ehp.118-a28.

7. A. A. Çerman et al., "Dietary Glycemic Factors, Insulin Resistance, and Adiponectin Levels in Acne Vulgaris," *Journal of the American Academy of Dermatology* 75, no. 1 (July 2016): 155–62, https://doi.org/10.1016/j.jaad.2016.02.1220.

8. J. Burris et al., "Differences in Dietary Glycemic Load and Hormones in New York City Adults with No and Moderate/Severe Acne," *Journal of the Academy of Nutrition and Dietetics* 117, no. 9 (September 2017): 1375–83, https://doi.org/10.1016/j.jand.2017.03.024.

9. R. Smith, "A Pilot Study to Determine the Short-Term Effects of a Low Glycemic Load Diet on Hormonal Markers of Acne: A Nonrandomized, Parallel, Controlled Feeding Trial," *Molecular Nutrition & Food Research* 52, no. 6 (June 2008): 718–26, https://doi.org/10.1002/mnfr.200700307.

10. G. Rosenblat et al., "Polyhydroxylated Fatty Alcohols Derived from Avocado Suppress Inflammatory Response and Provide Non-Sunscreen Protection Against UV-Induced Damage in Skin Cells," *Archives of Dermatological Research* 303, no. 4 (May 2011): 239–46, https://doi.org/10.1007/s00403-010-1088-6, erratum in *Archives of Dermatological Research* 303, no. 4 (May 2011): 299, http://dx.doi.org/10.1007/s00403-011-1139-7.

11. C. Nagata et al., "Association of Dietary Fat, Vegetables and Antioxidant Micronutrients with Skin Ageing in Japanese Women," *British Journal of Nutrition* 103, no. 10 (May 2010): 1493–8, https://doi.org/10.1017/S0007114509993461.

12. R. L. Roberts, J. Green, and B. Lewis, "Lutein and Zeaxanthin in Eye and Skin Health," *Clinics in Dermatology* 27, no. 2 (March–April 2009): 195–201, https://doi.org/10.1016/j.clindermatol.2008.01.011.

13. W. J. Cunliffe, "Unacceptable Side-Effects of Oral Zinc Sulphate in the Treatment of Acne Vulgaris," *British Journal of Dermatology* 101, no. 3 (September 1979): 363, https://doi.org/10.1111/j.1365-2133.1979.tb05636.x.

14. K. E. Sharquie, R. A. Najim, and H. N. Al-Salman, "Oral Zinc Sulfate in the Treatment of Rosacea: A Double-Blind, Placebo-Controlled Study," *International Journal of Dermatology* 45, no. 7 (July 2006): 857–61.

15. M. Gupta et al., "Zinc Therapy in Dermatology: A Review," *Dermatology Research and Practice* 2014 (July 2014): 709152, https://doi.org/10.1155/2014/709152.

16. D. De Mel and C. Suphioglu, "Fishy Business: Effect of Omega-3 Fatty Acids on Zinc Transporters and Free Zinc Availability in Human Neuronal Cells," *Nutrients* 6, no. 8 (August 2014): 3245–58, https://doi.org/10.3390/nu6083245.

17. H. S. Black and L. E. Rhodes, "Potential Benefits of Omega-3 Fatty Acids in Non-Melanoma Skin Cancer," *Journal of Clinical Medicine* 5, no. 2 (2016): 23, https://doi.org/10.3390/jcm5020023.

18. J. A. Evans and E. J. Johnson, "The Role of Phytonutrients in Skin Health," *Nutrients* 2, no. 8 (August 2010): 903–28, https://doi.org/10.3390/nu2080903.

19. Y. Shao et al., "Molecular Basis of Retinol Anti-Ageing Properties in Naturally Aged Human Skin in Vivo," *International Journal of Cosmetic Science* 39, no. 1 (February 2017): 56–65, https://doi.org/10.1111/ics.12348.

20. J. L. Arbiser et al., "Selenium Unmasks Protective Iron Armor: A Possible Defense Against Cutaneous Inflammation and Cancer," *Biochimica et Biophysica Acta (BBA): General Subjects* 1862, no. 11 (November 2018): 2518–27, https://doi.org/10.1016/j.bbagen.2018.05.018.

21. E. Weiss and R. Katta, "Diet and Rosacea: The Role of Dietary Change in the Management of Rosacea," *Dermatology Practical & Conceptual* 7, no. 4 (October 2017): 31–7, https://doi.org/10.5826/dpc.0704a08.

22. T. H. Zhu, "Epithelial Barrier Dysfunctions in Atopic Dermatitis: A Skin-Gut-Lung Model Linking Microbiome Alteration and Immune Dysregulation," *British Journal of Dermatology* 179, no. 3 (September 2018): 570–81, https://doi.org/10.1111/bjd.16734.

23. M. J. Bull and N. T. Plummer, "Part 1: The Human Gut Microbiome in Health and Disease," *Integrative Medicine* (Encinitas) 13, no. 6 (December 2014): 17–22.

24. A. Parodi et al., "Small Intestinal Bacterial Overgrowth in Rosacea: Clinical Effectiveness of Its Eradication," *Clinical Gastroenterology and Hepatology* 6, no. 7 (July 2008): 759–64, https://doi.org/10.1016/j.cgh.2008.02.054; H. Song et al., "*Faecalibacterium prausnitzii* Subspecies-Level Dysbiosis in the Human Gut Microbiome Underlying Atopic Dermatitis," *Journal of Allergy and Clinical Immunology* 137, no. 3 (March 2016): 852–60, https://doi.org/10.1016/j.jaci.2015.08.021.

25. G. Fabbrocini et al., "Supplementation with *Lactobacillus rhamnosus* SP1 Normalises Skin Expression of Genes Implicated in Insulin Signalling and Improves Adult Acne," *Beneficial Microbes* 7, no. 5 (November 2016): 625–30, https://doi.org/10.3920/BM2016.0089; Y. Saito et al., "Effects of Intake of Lactobacillus casei subsp. casei 327 on Skin Conditions: A Randomized, Double-Blind, Placebo-Controlled, Parallel-Group Study in Women," *Bioscience of Microbiota, Food and Health* 36, no. 3 (2017): 111–20, https://doi.org/10.12938/bmfh.16-031.

26. E. C. S. Bostock, K. C. Kirkby, and B. V. M. Taylor, "The Current Status of the Ketogenic Diet in Psychiatry," *Frontiers in Psychiatry* 8(March 2017): 43, https://doi.org/10.3389/fpsyt.2017.00043.

27. M. van de Wouw et al., "Short-Chain Fatty Acids: Microbial Metabolites that Alleviate Stress-Induced Brain-Gut Axis Alterations," *The Journal of Physiology* 596, no. 20 (October 2018): 4923-44, https://doi.org/10.1113/JP276431.

28. A. M. Taylor and H. D. Holscher, "A Review of Dietary and Microbial Connections to Depression, Anxiety, and Stress," *Nutritional Neuroscience* 9 (July 2018):1–14, https://doi.org/10.1080/1028415X.2018.1493808.

29. M. Torabi et al., "Effects of Nano and Conventional Zinc Oxide on Anxiety-Like Behavior in Male Rats," *Indian Journal of Pharmacology* 45, no. 5 (September–October 2013): 508–12, https://doi.org/10.4103/0253-7613.117784.

30. J. K. Kiecolt-Glaser et al., "Omega-3 Supplementation Lowers Inflammation and Anxiety in Medical Students: A Randomized Controlled Trial," *Brain, Behavior, and Immunity* 25, no. 8 (November 2011): 1725–34, https://doi.org/10.1016/j.bbi.2011.07.229.

31. M. R. Hilimire, J. E. DeVylder, and C. A. Forestell, "Fermented Foods, Neuroticism, and Social Anxiety: An Interaction Model," *Psychiatry Research* 228, no. 2 (August 2015): 203–8, https://doi.org/10.1016/j.psychres.2015.04.023.

32. T. C. Ooi et al., "Relationship between Testosterone, Estradiol, and Circulating PCSK9: Cross-Sectional and Interventional Studies in Humans," *Clinica Chimica Acta* 446 (June 2015): 97–104, https://doi.org/10.1016/j.cca.2015.03.036.

33. M. R. Mogarekar and S. K. Kulkarni, "Small Dense Low Density Lipoprotein Cholesterol, Paraoxonase 1 and Lipid Profile in Postmenopausal Women: Quality or Quantity?" *Archives of Medical Research* 46, no. 7 (October 2015): 534–38, https://doi.org/10.1016/j.arcmed.2015.08.007.

34. "Editorial Board," *Endocrinology* 156, no. 5 (May 2015): 1A, https://academic.oup.com/endo/issue/156/5.

35. C. Napoli and L. J. Ignarro, "Nitric Oxide and Pathogenic Mechanisms Involved in the Development of Vascular Diseases," *Archives of Pharmacal Research* 32, no. 8 (August 2009), 1103–08, https://doi.org/10.1007/s12272-009-1801-1.

36. E. Nevzati et al., "Estrogen Induces Nitric Oxide Production via Nitric Oxide Synthase Activation in Endothelial Cells," in *Neurovascular Events after Subarachnoid Hemorrhage,* edited by J. Fandino et al., *Acta Neurochirurgica Supplement* 120, (Switzerland: Springer, Cham, 2015) 141–45, https://doi.org/10.1007/978-3-319-04981-6_24.

37. A. Pinto et al., "Anti-Oxidant and Anti-Inflammatory Activity of Ketogenic Diet: New Perspectives for Neuroprotection in Alzheimer's Disease," *Antioxidants* 7, no. 5 (April 2018): 63, https://doi.org/:10.3390/antiox7050063.

38. C. Boots and E. Jungheim, "Inflammation and Human Ovarian Follicular Dynamics," *Seminars in Reproductive Medicine* 33, no. 4 (July 2015): 270–5, https://doi.org/10.1055/s-0035-1554928.

39. J. C. Mavropoulos et al., "The effects of a low-carbohydrate, ketogenic diet on the polycystic ovary syndrome: a pilot study," *Journal of Nutrition and Metabolism* 2, (December 2005): 35, https://doi.org/ 10.1186/1743-7075-2-35.

40. J. Wilson et al., "The Effects of Ketogenic Dieting on Body Composition, Strength, Power, and Hormonal Profiles in Resistance Training Males," *Journal of Strength and Conditioning Research,* (October 2017), https://doi.org/10.1519/JSC.0000000000001935.

41. Y. Qi et al., "Adiponectin Acts in the Brain to Decrease Body Weight," *Nature Medicine* 10, no. 5 (April 2004): 524–29, https://doi.org/10.1038/nm1029.

42. A. Achari and S. Jain, "Adiponectin, a Therapeutic Target for Obesity, Diabetes, and Endothelial Dysfunction," *International Journal of Molecular Sciences* 18, no. 6 (June 2017): 1321, https://doi.org/10.3390/ijms18061321.

43. L. E. Norris et al., "Comparison of Dietary Conjugated Linoleic Acid with Safflower Oil on Body Composition in Obese Postmenopausal Women with Type 2 Diabetes Mellitus," *The American Journal of Clinical Nutrition* 90, no. 3 (September 2009): 468–76, https://doi.org/10.3945/ajcn.2008.27371.

44. R. H. Lustig et al., "Obesity, Leptin Resistance, and the Effects of Insulin reduction," *International Journal of Obesity* 28, no. 10 (October 2004):1344–8, https://doi.org/10.1038/sj.ijo.0802753.

45. M. Wohlers et al., "Effect of Fish or Soybean Oil-Rich Diets on Bradykinin, Kallikrein, Nitric Oxide, Leptin, Corticosterone, and Macrophages in Carrageenan Stimulated Rats," *Inflammation* 29, no. 2–3 (June 2005): 81-9, https://doi.org/10.1007/s10753-006-9002-2.

46. K. Spiegel et al., "Leptin Levels Are Dependent on Sleep Duration: Relationships with Sympathovagal Balance, Carbohydrate Regulation, Cortisol, and Thyrotropin," *The Journal of Clinical Endocrinology & Metabolism* 89, no. 11 (November 2004): 5762–71, https://doi.org/10.1210/jc.2004-1003.

47. M. Daghestani, "A Preprandial and Postprandial Plasma Levels of Ghrelin Hormone in Lean, Overweight, and Obese Saudi females," *Journal of King Saud University–Science* 21, no. 2 (July 2009): 119–24, https://doi.org/10.1016/j.jksus.2009.05.001.

48. Wohlers et al., "Effect of Fish or Soybean Oil-Rich Diets on Bradykinin, Kallikrein, Nitric Oxide, Leptin, Corticosterone, and Macrophages in Carrageenan Stimulated Rats," 81-9.

49. R. C. Fernandez et al., "Fixed or Rotating Night Shift Work Undertaken by Women: Implications for Fertility and Miscarriage," *Seminars in Reproductive Medicine* 32, no. 2 (March 2016): 74–82, https://doi.org/10.1055/s-0036-1571354.

50. J. M. Baker, L. Al-Nakkash, and M. M. Herbst-Kralovetz, "Estrogen–Gut Microbiome Axis: Physiological and Clinical Implications," *Maturitas* 103 (September 2017): 45–53, https://doi.org/10.1016/j.maturitas.2017.06.025.

51. L. Baker et al., "The Role of Estrogen in Cardiovascular Disease," *Journal of Surgical Research* 115, no. 2 (December 2003): 325–44, https://doi.org/ 10.1016/ s0022-4804(03)00215-4.

52. F. Lizcano and G. Guzmán, "Estrogen Deficiency and the Origin of Obesity during Menopause," *Biomed Research International* 2014 (2014): 757461, https:// doi.org/10.1155/2014/757461.

53. L. Lindheim et al., "Alterations in Gut Microbiome Composition and Barrier Function Are Associated with Reproductive and Metabolic Defects in Women with Polycystic Ovary Syndrome (PCOS): A Pilot Study," *PLoS One* 12, no. 1 (January 2017): e0168390, https://doi.org/10.1371/journal.pone.0168390.

54. Baker, *Maturitas* 103: 45–53.

55. T. C. Birdsall, "5-Hydroxytryptophan: a Clinically-Effective Serotonin Precursor," *Alternative Medicine Review* 3, no. 4 (August 1998): 271–80.

56. Y. Yang et al., "Melatonin as Potential Targets for Delaying Ovarian Aging," *Current Drug Targets* 20, no. 1 (2019): 16–28, https://doi.org/10.2174/1389450119 666180828144843.

# Chapter 5

1. Popkin, D'Anci, and Rosenberg, "Water, Hydration and Health," 439–58.

2. X. Zhang et al., "Cruciferous Vegetable Consumption Is Associated with a Reduced Risk of Total and Cardiovascular Disease Mortality," *The American Journal of Clinical Nutrition* 94, no. 1 (July 2011): 240–6, https://doi.org/10.3945/ ajcn.110.009340.

3. C. E. Guerrero-Beltrán et al., "Protective Effect of Sulforaphane Against Oxidative Stress: Recent Advances," *Experimental and Toxicologic Pathology* 64, no. 5 (July 2012): 503–8, https://doi.org/10.1016/j.etp.2010.11.005.

4. D. L. Folkard et al., "Effect of Sulforaphane on NOD2 via NF-κB: Implications for Crohn's disease," *Journal of Inflammation* 12 (January 2015): 6, https://doi .org/10.1186/s12950-015-0051-x.

5. K. J. Royston and T. O. Tollefsbol, "The Epigenetic Impact of Cruciferous Vegetables on Cancer Prevention," *Current Pharmacology Reports* 1, no. 1 (February 2015): 46–51, https://doi.org/ 10.1007/s40495-014-0003-9.

6. H. B. Sowbhagya, "Chemistry, Technology, and Nutraceutical Functions of Celery (*Apium graveolens* L.): An Overview," Critical Reviews in Food Science and Nutrition 54, no. 3 (2013): 389–98, https://doi.org/10.1080/10408398.2011.586740.

7. L. M. Sanders and S. H. Zeisel, "Choline: Dietary Requirements and Role in Brain Development," *Nutrition Today* 42, no. 4 (July–August 2007): 181–6, https://doi.org/10.1097/01.NT.0000286155.55343.fa.

8. National Cancer Institute, "Cruciferious Vegetables and Cancer Prevention," Reviewed June 7, 2012, http://www.cancer.gov/cancertopics/causes-prevention/risk/diet/cruciferous-vegetables-fact-sheet.

9. C. P. Bondonno et al., "Flavonoid-Rich Apples and Nitrate-Rich Spinach Augment Nitric Oxide Status and Improve Endothelial Function in Healthy Men and Women: A Randomized Controlled Trial," *Free Radical Biology and Medicine* 52, no. 1 (January 2012): 95–102, https://doi.org/10.1016/j.freeradbiomed.2011.09.028.

10. MedlinePlus, "Manganese," U.S. National Library of Medicine, Last reviewed May 31, 2019, http://www.nlm.nih.gov/medlineplus/druginfo/natural/182.html.

11. J. B. Wang et al., "Dietary Components and Risk of Total, Cancer and Cardiovascular Disease Mortality in the Linxian Nutrition Intervention Trials Cohort in China," *Scientific Reports* 6 (March 2016): 22619, https://doi.org/10.1038/srep22619.

12. J. Fiedor and K. Burda, "Potential Role of Carotenoids as Antioxidants in Human Health and Disease," *Nutrients* 6, no. 2 (January 2014): 466–88, https://doi.org/10.3390/nu6020466.

13. P. Y. Wang et al., "Higher Intake of Fruits, Vegetables or Their Fiber Reduces the Risk of Type 2 Diabetes: A Meta-Analysis," *Journal of Diabetes Investigation* 7, no.1 (January 2016): 56–69, https://doi.org/10.1111/jdi.12376.

14. O. Azarenko, M. A. Jordan, and L. Wilson, "Erucin, the Major Isothiocyanate in Arugula (*Eruca sativa*), Inhibits Proliferation of MCF7 Tumor Cells by Suppressing Microtubule Dynamics," *PLoS One* 9 no. 6, (June 2014): e100599, https://doi.org/10.1371/journal.pone.0100599.

15. F. E. Wirngo, M. N. Lambert, and P. B. Jeppesen, "The Physiological Effects of Dandelion (*Taraxacum Officinale*) in Type 2 Diabetes," *The Review of Diabetic Studies* 13, no. 2–3 (2016): 113–31, https://doi.org/10.1900/RDS.2016.13.113.

16. A. J. Larson, J. D. Symons, and T. Jalili, "Therapeutic Potential of Quercetin to Decrease Blood Pressure: Review of Efficacy and Mechanisms," *Advances in Nutrition* 3, no. 1 (January 2012): 39–46, https://doi.org/10.3945/an.111.001271.

17. J. M. Calderón-Montaño et al., "A Review on the Dietary Flavonoid Kaempferol," *Mini Reviews in Medicinal Chemistry* 11, no. 4 (April 2011): 298–344.

18. J. Borlinghaus et al., "Allicin: Chemistry and Biological Properties," *Molecules* 19, no. 8 (August 2014): 12591–618, https://doi.org/10.3390/molecules190812591.

19. N. Mikami et al., "Reduction of HbA1c Levels by Fucoxanthin-Enriched Akamoku Oil Possibly Involves the Thrifty Allele of Uncoupling Protein 1 (UCP1): A Randomised Controlled Trial in Normal-Weight and Obese Japanese Adults," *Journal of Nutritional Science* 6 (February 2017): e5, https://doi.org/10.1017/jns.2017.1.

20. M. A. Gammone and N. D'Orazio, "Anti-obesity Activity of the Marine Carotenoid Fucoxanthin," *Marine Drugs* 13, no. 4 (April 2015): 2196–214, https://doi.org/10.3390/md13042196.

21. R. J. Turesky, "Heterocyclic Aromatic Amine Metabolism, DNA Adduct Formation, Mutagenesis, and Carcinogenesis," *Drug Metabolism Reviews* 34, no. 3 (July 2002): 625–50, https://doi.org/10.1081/DMR-120005665.

22. M. Sienkiewicz et al., "The Potential of Use Basil and Rosemary Essential Oils as Effective Antibacterial Agents," *Molecules* 18, no. 8 (August 2013): 9334–51, https://doi.org/10.3390/molecules18089334.

23. P. Suppakul et al., "Antimicrobial Properties of Basil and Its Possible Application in Food Packaging," *Journal of Agricultural and Food Chemistry* 51, no. 11 (May 2003): 3197–207.

24. N. Hayek, "Chocolate, Gut Microbiota, and Human Health," 11.

25. S. K. Verma, V. Jain, and S. S. Katewa, "Blood Pressure Lowering, Fibrinolysis Enhancing and Antioxidant Activities of Cardamom (*Elettaria cardamomum*)," *Indian Journal of Biochem and Biophysics* 46, no. 6 (December 2009): 503–6.

26. P. Vijayalakshmi, S. Thenmozhi, and P. Rajeswari, "The Evaluation of the Virulence Factors of Clinical Candida Isolates and the Anti-Biofilm Activity of *Elettaria cardamomum* Against Multi-Drug Resistant *Candida albicans*," *Current Medical Mycology* 2, no. 2 (June 2016): 8–15.

27. C. M. Kaefer and J. A. Milner, "Herbs and Spices in Cancer Prevention and Treatment," in *Herbal Medicine: Biomolecular and Clinical Aspects*, 2nd ed., edited by I. F. F. Benzie and S. Wachtel-Galor, (Boca Raton, FL: CRC Press, 2011).

28. B. Qin, K. S. Panickar, and R. A. Anderson, "Cinnamon: Potential Role in the Prevention of Insulin Resistance, Metabolic Syndrome, and Type 2 Diabetes," *Journal of Diabetes Science and Technology* 4, no.3 (May 2010): 685–93, https://doi.org/10.1177/193229681000400324.

29. Qin, "Cinnamon: Potential Role in the Prevention of Insulin Resistance, Metabolic Syndrome, and Type 2 Diabetes," 685–693.

30. J. Ravindran, S. Prasad, and B. B. Aggarwal, "Curcumin and Cancer Cells: How Many Ways Can Curry Kill Tumor Cells Selectively?" *The AAPS Journal* 11, no. 3 (September 2009): 495–510, https://doi.org/10.1208/s12248-009-9128-x.

31. P. Dulbecco and V. Savarino, "Therapeutic Potential of Curcumin in Digestive Diseases," *World Journal of Gastroenterology* 19, no. 48 (2013): 9256–270, https://doi.org/10.3748/wjg.v19.i48.9256.

32. E. Ernst and M. H. Pittler, "Efficacy of Ginger for Nausea and Vomiting: A Systematic Review of Randomized Clinical Trials," *British Journal of Anaesthesia* 84, no.3 (March 2000): 367–71, https://doi.org/10.1093/oxfordjournals.bja.a013442.

33. N. S. Mashhadi et al., "Anti-oxidative and Anti-inflammatory Effects of Ginger in Health and Physical Activity: Review of Current Evidence," *International Journal of Preventive Medicine* 4, Supplement 1 (April 2013): S36–S42.

34. Y. Teng et al., "Plant-Derived Exosomal MicroRNAs Shape the Gut Microbiota," *Cell Host & Microbe* 24, no. 5 (November 2018): 637–52, https://doi.org/10.1016/j.chom.2018.10.001.

35. J. Zhu et al., "Effects of Ginger (*Zingiber officinale Roscoe*) on Type 2 Diabetes Mellitus and Components of the Metabolic Syndrome: A Systematic Review and Meta-Analysis of Randomized Controlled Trials," *Evidence Based Complementary and Alternative Medicine* 2018 (2018): 5692962, https://doi.org/10.1155/2018/5692962.

36. I. Savini et al., *"Origanum Vulgare* Induces Apoptosis in Human Colon Cancer Caco2 Cells," *Nutrition and Cancer* 61, no. 3 (2009): 381–9, https://doi.org/10.1080/01635580802582769; Bonn University, "Salutary Pizza Spice: Oregano Helps Against Inflammations," *ScienceDaily* (June 2008), https://www.sciencedaily.com/releases/2008/06/080625093147.htm.

37. N. Leyva-López et al., "Essential Oils of Oregano: Biological Activity Beyond Their Antimicrobial Properties," *Molecules* 22, no. 6 (June 2017): 989, https://doi.org/10.3390/molecules22060989.

38. S. Sanati, B. M. Razavi, and H. Hosseinzadeh, "A Review of the Effects of *Capsicum annuum* L. and Its Constituent, Capsaicin, in Metabolic Syndrome," *Iranian Journal of Basic Medical Sciences* 21, no.5 (May 2018): 439–48, https://doi.org/10.22038/IJBMS.2018.25200.6238.

39. S. K. Panchal, E. Bliss, and L. Brown, "Capsaicin in Metabolic Syndrome," *Nutrients* 10, no. 5 (May 2018), https://doi.org/10.3390/nu10050630.

40. J. Moore, M. Yousef, and E. Tsiani, "Anticancer Effects of Rosemary (*Rosmarinus officinalis* L.) Extract and Rosemary Extract Polyphenols," *Nutrients* 8, no. 11 (November 2016): 731, https://doi.org/10.3390/nu8110731.

41. S. N. Ngo, D. B. Williams, and R. J. Head, "Rosemary and Cancer Prevention: Preclinical Perspectives," *Critical Reviews in Food Science and Nutrition* 51, no. 10 (December 2011): 946–54, https://doi.org/10.1080/10408398.2010.490883.

42. B. Salehi et al., "Thymol, Thyme, and Other Plant Sources: Health and Potential Uses," *Phytotherapy Research* 32, no. 9 (September 2018): 1688–1706, https://doi.org/10.1002/ptr.6109.

43. B. B. Aggarwal, "Targeting Inflammation-Induced Obesity and Metabolic Diseases by Curcumin and Other Nutraceuticals," *Annual Review of Nutrition* 30 (August 2010): 173–199, https://doi.org/10.1146/annurev.nutr.012809.104755.

44. H. O. Santos, A. A. Bueno, and J. F. Mota, "The Effect of Artichoke on Lipid Profiel: A Review of Possible Mechanisms of Action," *Pharmacological Research* 137 (November 2018): 170–8, https://doi.org/10.1016/j.phrs.2018.10.007.

45. E. N. Fissore et al., "A Study of the Effect of Dietary Fiber Fractions Obtained from Artichoke (*Cynara cardunculus* L. var. *scolymus*) on the Growth of Intestinal Bacteria Associated with Health," *Food & Function* 6, no. 5 (May 2015): 1667–74, https://doi.org/10.1039/c5fo00088b.

46. I. Mentel et al., "Content of Nutritive Components, Dietary Fibre and Energy Value of Artichoke Depending on the Variety," *Acta Scientiarum Polonorum Technologia Alimentaria* 11, no. 2 (April 2012): 201–7.

47. M. Ben Salem et al., "Pharmacological Studies of Artichoke Leaf Extract and Their Health Benefits," *Plant Foods for Human Nutrition* 70, no. 4 (December 2015): 441–53, https://doi.org/10.1007/s11130-015-0503-8.

48. A. Sahebkar et al., "Lipid-Lowering Activity of Artichoke Extracts: A Systematic Review and Meta-Analysis," *Critical Reviews in Food Science and Nutrition* 58, no. 15 (2018): 2549–2556, https://doi.org/10.1080/10408398.2017.1332572.

49. M. Nekohashi et al., "Luteolin and Quercetin Affect the Cholesterol Absorption Mediated by Epithelial Cholesterol Transporter Niemann-Pick C1-Like 1 in Caco-2 Cells and Rats," *PLoS One* 9, no. 5 (May 2014): e97901, https://doi.org/10.1371/journal.pone.0097901.

50. V. L. Fulgoni III, M. Dreher, and A. J. Davenport, "Avocado Consumption Is Associated with Better Diet Quality and Nutrient Intake, and Lower Metabolic Syndrome Risk in US Adults: Results from the National Health and Nutrition Examination Survey (NHANES) 2001–2008," *Nutrition Journal* 12 (January 2013): 1, https://doi.org/10.1186/1475-2891-12-1.

51. A. Cassidy, "Berry Anthocyanin Intake and Cardiovascular Health," *Molecular Aspects of Medicine* 61 (June 2018): 76–82, https://doi.org/10.1016/j.mam.2017.05.002.

52. C. Ceci et al., "Experimental Evidence of the Antitumor, Antimetastatic and Antiangiogenic Activity of Ellagic Acid," *Nutrients* 10, no.11 (November 2018): 1756, https://doi.org/10.3390/nu10111756.

53. L. T. Toscano et al., "Chia Flour Supplementation Reduces Blood Pressure in Hypertensive Subjects," *Plant Foods for Human Nutrition* 69, no. 4 (December 2014): 392–8, https://doi.org/10.1007/s11130-014-0452-7.

54. H. Ho et al., "Effect of Whole and Ground Salba Seeds (*Salvia Hispanica* L.) on Postprandial Glycemia in Healthy Volunteers: A Randomized Controlled, Dose-Response Trial," *European Journal of Clinical Nutrition* 67, no. 7 (July 2013): 786–8, https://doi.org/10.1038/ejcn.2013.103.

55. K. K. Singh et al., "Flaxseed: A Potential Source of Food, Feed and Fiber," *Critical Reviews in Food Science and Nutrition* 51, no. 3 (March 2011): 210–22, https://doi.org/10.1080/10408390903537241.

56. A. Akrami et al., "Comparison of the Effects of Flaxseed Oil and Sunflower Seed Oil Consumption on Serum Glucose, Lipid Profile, Blood Pressure, and Lipid Peroxidation in Patients with Metabolic Syndrome," *Journal of Clinical Lipidology* 12, no. 1 (January–February 2018): 70–77, https://doi.org/10.1016/j.jacl.2017.11.004.

57. D. J. Jenkins et al., "Almonds Decrease Postprandial Glycemia, Insulinemia, and Oxidative Damage in Healthy Individuals," *The Journal of Nutrition* 136, no. 12 (December 2006): 2987–92, https://doi.org/ 10.1093/jn/136.12.2987.

58. I. D. Platt et al., "Postprandial Effects of Almond Consumption on Human Osteoclast Precursors—an Ex Vivo Study," *Metabolism* 60, no. 7 (July 2011): 923–9, https://doi.org/10.1016/j.metabol.2010.08.012.

59. C. Berryman, J. Fleming, and P. Kris-Etherton, "Inclusion of Almonds in a Cholesterol-Lowering Diet Improves Plasma HDL Subspecies and Cholesterol Efflux to Serum in Normal-Weight Individuals with Elevated LDL Cholesterol," *The Journal of Nutrition* 147, no. 8 (August 2017): 1517–23, https://doi.org/10.3945/jn.116.245126.

60. S. Blanco Mejia et al., "Effect of Tree Nuts on Metabolic Syndrome Criteria: A Systematic Review and Meta-Analysis of Randomised Controlled Trials," *BMJ Open* 4, no. 7 (2014): e004660, https://doi.org/10.1136/bmjopen-2013-004660.

61. A. M. Tindall et al., "Tree Nut Consumption and Adipose Tissue Mass: Mechanisms of Action," *Current Developments in Nutrition* 2, no. 11 (August 2018): nzy069, https://doi.org/10.1093/cdn/nzy069.

62. C. Hudthagosol et al., "Pecans Acutely Increase Plasma Postprandial Antioxidant Capacity and Catechins and Decrease LDL Oxidation in Humans," *The Journal of Nutrition* 141, no. 1 (2010): 56–62, https://doi.org/10.3945/jn.110.121269.

63. M. Gossell-Williams et al., "Improvement in HDL Cholesterol in Postmenopausal Women Supplemented with Pumpkin Seed Oil: Pilot Study," *Climacteric* 14, no. 5 (October 2011): 558–64, https://doi.org/10.3109/13697137.2011.563882.

64. K. Richmond et al., "Markers of Cardiovascular Risk in Postmenopausal Women with Type 2 Diabetes Are Improved by the Daily Consumption of Almonds or Sunflower Kernels: A Feeding Study," *ISRN Nutrition* 2013 (December 2012): 626414, https://doi.org/10.5402/2013/626414.

65. D. Hayes et al., "Walnuts *(Juglans regia)* Chemical Composition and Research in Human Health," *Critical Reviews in Food Science and Nutrition* 56, no. 8 (June 2016): 1231–41, https://doi.org/10.1080/10408398.2012.760516.

66. H. Holscher et al., "Walnut Consumption Alters the Gastrointestinal Microbiota, Microbially Derived Secondary Bile Acids, and Health Markers in Healthy Adults: A Randomized Controlled Trial," *The Journal of Nutrition* 148, no. 6 (June 2018): 861–7, https://doi.org/10.1093/jn/nxy004.

67. T. Kondo et al., "Vinegar Intake Reduces Body Weight, Body Fat Mass, and Serum Triglyceride Levels in Obese Japanese Subjects," *Bioscience, Biotechnology, and Biochemistry* 73, no. 8 (August 2009): 1837–43.

68. J. Lim, C. J. Henry, and S. Haldar, "Vinegar as a Functional Ingredient to Improve Postprandial Glycemic Control-Human Intervention Findings and Molecular Mechanisms," *Molecular Nutrition & Food Research* 60, no. 8 (August 2016): 1837–49, https://doi.org/10.1002/mnfr.201600121.

69. D. Yagnik, V. Serafin, A. J. Shah, "Antimicrobial Activity of Apple Cider Vinegar Against *Escherichia coli, Staphylococcus aureus* and *Candida albicans*; Downregulating Cytokine and Microbial Protein Expression," *Scientific Reports* 8, no. 1 (January 2018): 1732, https://doi.org/10.1038/s41598-017-18618-x.

70. Y. Jiang et al., "Cruciferous Vegetable Intake Is Inversely Correlated with Circulating Levels of Proinflammatory Markers in Women," *Journal of the Academy of Nutrition and Dietetics* 114, no. 5 (May 2014): 700–8.e2, https://doi.org/10.1016/j.jand.2013.12.019.

71. R. T. Ras, J. M. Geleijnse, E. A. Trautwein, "LDL-Cholesterol-Lowering Effect of Plant Sterols and Stanols Across Different Dose Ranges: A Meta-Analysis of Randomised Controlled Studies," *British Journal of Nutrition* 112, no. 2 (July 2014): 214–9, https://doi.org/10.1017/S0007114514000750.

72. H. Wang et al., "Yogurt Consumption Is Associated with Better Diet Quality and Metabolic Profile in American Men and Women," *Nutrition Research* 33, no. 1 (January 2013): 18–26, https://doi.org/10.1016/j.nutres.2012.11.009.

73. Jun Zou et al., "Fiber-Mediated Nourishment of Gut Microbiota Protects against Diet-Induced Obesity by Restoring IL-22-Mediated Colonic Health," *Cell Host & Microbe* 23, no. 1 (January 2018): 41–53.E4, https://doi.org/10.1016/j.chom.2017.11.003.

74. Z. Madani et al., "Dietary Sardine Protein Lowers Insulin Resistance, Leptin and TNF-α and Beneficially Affects Adipose Tissue Oxidative Stress in Rats with Fructose-Induced Metabolic Syndrome," *International Journal of Molecular Medicine* 29, no. 2 (February 2012): 311–8, https://doi.org/10.3892/ijmm.2011.836.

75. A. S. Prasad, "Discovery of Human Zinc Deficiency: Its Impact on Human Health and Disease," *Advances in Nutrition* 4, no. 2 (March 2013): 176–90, https://doi.org/10.3945/an.112.003210.

76. E. R. De Oliveira e Silva et al., "Effects of Shrimp Consumption on Plasma Lipoproteins," *The American Journal of Clinical Nutrition* 64, no. 5 (November 1996): 712–7, https://doi.org/10.1093/ajcn/64.5.712.

77. National Institutes of Health, "Vitamin B12: Fact Sheet for Professionals," Updated November 29, 2018, https://ods.od.nih.gov/factsheets/VitaminB12 -HealthProfessional/.

78. T. Iwamoto et al., "Inhibition of Low-Density Lipoprotein Oxidation by Astaxanthin," *Journal of Atherosclerosis Thrombosis* 7, no. 4 (2000): 216–22, https://doi.org/ 10.5551/jat1994.7.216.

79. L. Qi et al., "Independent and Synergistic Associations of Biomarkers of Vitamin D Status with Risk of Coronary Heart Disease," *Arterioscleris, Thrombosis, and Vascular Biology* 37, no. 11 (November 2017): 2204–12, https://doi.org/10.1161/ ATVBAHA.117.309548.

80. S. Pilz et al., "Association of Vitamin D Deficiency with Heart Failure and Sudden Cardiac Death in a Large Cross-Sectional Study of Patients Referred for Coronary Angiography," *The Journal of Clinical Endocrinology & Metabolism* 93, no. 10 (October 2008): 3927–35, https://doi.org/10.1210/jc.2008-0784.

81. M. Dreher and A. Davenport, "Hass Avocado Composition and Potential Health Effects," *Critical Reviews in Food Science and Nutrition* 53, no. 7 (2013): 738–750, https://doi.org/10.1080/10408398.2011.556759.

82. A. Basu, S. Devaraj, and I. Jialal, "Dietary Factors that Promote or Retard Inflammation," *Arterioscleris, Thrombosis, and Vascular Biology* 26, no. 5 (May 2006): 995–1001, https://doi.org/10.1161/01.ATV.0000214295.86079.d1.

83. J. A. Menendez et al., "Oleic Acid, the Main Monounsaturated Fatty Acid of Olive Oil, Suppresses Her-2/neu (erbB-2) Expression and Synergistically Enhances the Growth Inhibitory Effects of Trastuzumab (Herceptin) in Breast Cancer Cells with Her-2/neu Oncogene Amplification," *Annals of Oncology* 16, no. 3 (March 2005): 359–71.

84. J. J. Kabara et al., "Fatty Acids and Derivatives as Antimicrobial Agents," *Antimicrobial Agents and Chemotherapy* 2, no: 1 (1972): 23–28, https://doi.org/ 10.1128/aac.2.1.23.

85. D. A. Cardoso et al., "A Coconut Extra Virgin Oil-Rich Diet Increases HDL Cholesterol and Decreases Waist Circumference and Body Mass in Coronary Artery Disease Patients," *Nutrición Hospitalaria* 32, no. 5 (November 2015): 2144–52, https://doi.org/10.3305/nh.2015.32.5.9642.

86. L. Schwingshackl and G. Hoffmann, "Monounsaturated Fatty Acids, Olive Oil and Health Status: A Systematic Review and Meta-Analysis of Cohort Studies," *Lipids in Health and Disease* 13 (October 2014): 154, https://doi.org/10.1186/ 1476-511X-13-154.

87. L. Lucas, A. Russell, and R. Keast, "Molecular Mechanisms of Inflammation. Anti-inflammatory Benefits of Virgin Olive Oil and the Phenolic Compound Oleocanthal," *Current Pharmaceutical Design* 17, no. 8 (2011): 754–68, https:// doi.org/ 10.2174/138161211795428911.

88. D. Sankar et al., "Effect of Sesame Oil on Diuretics or Beta-Blockers in the Modulation of Blood Pressure, Anthropometry, Lipid Profile, and Redox Status," *Yale Journal of Biology and Medicine* 79, no. 1 (March 2006): 19–26.

89. C. Chaicharoenpong and A. Petsom. "Use of Tea (*Camellia oleifera* Abel.) Seeds in human Health," in *Nuts & Seeds in Health and Disease Prevention*, 1st ed., ed. V. R. Preedy, R. R. Watson, V. B. Patel (London, Burlington, San Diego: Academic Press 2011), 1115–22.

90. B. E. Wolfe et al., "Cheese Rind Communities Provide Tractable Systems for In Situ and In Vitro Studies of Microbial Diversity," *Cell* 158, no. 2 (July 2014): 422, https://doi.org/10.1016/j.cell.2014.05.041.

91. Z. Radulović et al., "Survival of Spray-Dried and Free-Cells of Potential Probiotic *Lactobacillus plantarum* 564 in Soft Goat Cheese," *Animal Science Journal* 88, no. 11 (November 2017): 1849–54. https://doi.org/10.1111/asj.12802.

92. S. Jianqin et al., "Effects of milk containing only A2 beta casein versus milk containing both A1 and A2 beta casein proteins on gastrointestinal physiology, symptoms of discomfort, and cognitive behavior of people with self-reported intolerance to traditional cows' milk," *Nutrition Journal* 15, no. 35 (April 2016), https://doi.org/10.1186/s12937-016-0147-z.

93. N. Castro-Webb, E. A. Ruiz-Narváez, and H. Campos, "Cross-Sectional Study of Conjugated Linoleic Acid in Adipose Tissue and Risk of Diabetes," *The American Journal of Clinical Nutrition* 96, no. 1 (July 2012): 175–81, https://doi.org/10.3945/ajcn.111.011858.

94. H. Blankson et al., "Conjugated Linoleic Acid Reduces Body Fat Mass in Overweight and Obese Humans," *The Journal of Nutrition* 130, no. 12 (December 2000): 2943–8, https://doi.org/10.1093/jn/130.12.2943.

95. J. E. Kanter et al., "10,12 Conjugated Linoleic Acid-Driven Weight Loss Is Protective against Atherosclerosis in Mice and Is Associated with Alternative Macrophage Enrichment in Perivascular Adipose Tissue," *Nutrients* 10, no. 10 (October 2018): 1416, https://doi.org/10.3390/nu10101416.

96. H. Zheng et al., "Metabolomics Investigation to Shed Light on Cheese as a Possible Piece in the French Paradox Puzzle," *Journal of Agricultural and Food Chemistry* 63, no. 10 (March 2015): 2830–9, https://doi.org/10.1021/jf505878a.

97. J. K. Lorenzen and A. Astrup, "Dairy calcium intake modifies responsiveness of fat metabolism and blood lipids to a high-fat diet," *British Journal of Nutrition* 105, no. 12 (June 2011): 1823–31, https://doi.org/10.1017/S0007114510005581.

98. C. Richard et al., "Impact of Egg Consumption on Cardiovascular Risk Factors in Individuals with Type 2 Diabetes and at Risk for Developing Diabetes: A Systematic Review of Randomized Nutritional Intervention Studies," *Canadian Journal of Diabetes* 41, no. 4 (August 2017): 453–63, https://doi.org/10.1016/j.jcjd.2016.12.002.

99. N. R. Fuller et al., "Effect of a High-Egg Diet on Cardiometabolic Risk Factors in People with Type 2 Diabetes: The Diabetes and Egg (DIABEGG) Study—Randomized Weight-Loss and Follow-Up Phase," *The American Journal of Clinical Nutrition* 107, no. 6 (June 2018): 921–31, https://doi.org/10.1093/ajcn/nqy048.

100. D. M. DiMarco et al., "Intake of up to 3 Eggs/Day Increases HDL Cholesterol and Plasma Choline while Plasma Trimethylamine-N-oxide Is Unchanged in a Healthy Population," *Lipids* 52, no. 3 (March 2017): 255–63, https://doi.org/10.1007/s11745-017-4230-9.

101. Y. Suzuki et al., "Antidiabetic effect of long-term supplementation with *Siraitia grosvenori* on the spontaneously diabetic Goto–Kakizaki rat," *British Journal of Nutrition* 97, no. 4 (April 2007): 770–75, https://doi.org/10.1017/S0007114507381300.

102. W. J. Chen et al., "The antioxidant activities of natural sweeteners, mogrosides, from fruits of *Siraitia grosvenori*," *International Journal of Food Sciences and Nutrition* 58, no. 7 (July 2009): 548–56, https://doi.org/10.1080/09637480701336360.

103. X. Y. Qi et al., "Mogrosides extract from *Siraitia grosvenori* scavenges free radicals in vitro and lowers oxidative stress, serum glucose, and lipid levels in alloxan-induced diabetic mice," *Nutrition Research* 28, no. 4 (April 2008): 278–84, https://doi.org/10.1016/j.nutres.2008.02.008.

104. K. Philippaert et al., "Steviol glycosides enhance pancreatic beta-cell function and taste sensation by potentiation of TRPM5 channel activity," *Nature Communications* 8 (March 2017), https://doi.org/10.1038/NCOMMS14733.

105. M. Hiele et al., "Metabolism of erythritol in humans: Comparison with glucose and lactitol," *British Journal of Nutrition* 69, no. 1 (January 1993): 169–76, https://doi.org/10.1079/BJN19930019.

106. M. Grembecka, "Sugar alcohols—their role in the modern world of sweeteners: a review," *European Food Research and Technology* 241, no. 1 (July 2015): 1–14, https://doi.org/10.1007/s00217-015-2437-7.

107. E. N. Ponnampalam, N. J. Mann, and A. J. Sinclair, "Effect of Feeding Systems on Omega-3 Fatty Acids, Conjugated Linoleic Acid and Trans Fatty Acids in Australian Beef Cuts: Potential Impact on Human Health," *Asia Pacific Journal of Clinical Nutrition* 15, no. 1 (2006): 21–9.

108. O. P. Wójcik et al., "Serum Taurine and Risk of Coronary Heart Disease: A Prospective, Nested Case-Control Study," *European Journal of Nutrition* 52, no. 1 (February 2013): 169–78, https://doi.org/10.1007/s00394-011-0300-6.

109. M. Meyer-Ficca and J. B. Kirkland, "Niacin," *Advances in Nutrition: An International Review Journal* 7, no. 3 (May 2016): 556–8, https://doi.org/10.3945/an.115.011239.

110. D. Gill et al., "The Effect of Iron Status on Risk of Coronary Artery Disease: A Mendelian Randomization Study-Brief Report," *Arteriosclerosis, Thrombosis, and Vascular Biology* 37, no. 9 (September 2017): 1788–92, https://doi.org/10.1161/ATVBAHA.117.309757.

111. B. Y. Silber and J. A. Schmitt, "Effects of Tryptophan Loading on Human Cognition, Mood, and Sleep," *Neuroscience & Biobehavioral Reviews* 34, no. 3 (February 2010): 387–407, https://doi.org/10.1016/j.neubiorev.2009.08.005.

# Chapter 6

1.  M. F. Holick and T. C. Chen, "Vitamin D Deficiency: A Worldwide Problem with Health Consequences," *The American Journal of Clinical Nutrition* 87, no. 4 (April 2008): 1080S–6S, https://doi.org/10.1093/ajcn/87.4.1080S.

2.  Institute of Medicine (US) Committee to Review Dietary Reference Intakes for Vitamin D and Calcium, "Overview of Vitamin D," *Dietary Reference Intakes for Calcium and Vitamin D*, ed. A. C. Ross et al. (Washington, DC: National Academies Press, 2011), 75–111, https://www.ncbi.nlm.nih.gov/books/NBK56061.

3.  K. Y. Forrest and W. L. Stuhldreher, "Prevalence and Correlates of Vitamin D Deficiency in US Adults," *Nutrition Research* 31, no. 1 (January 2011): 48–54.

4.  P. Pludowski et al., "Vitamin D Supplementation Guidelines," *The Journal of Steroid Biochemistry and Molecular Biology* 175 (January 2018): 125–35, https://doi.org/10.1016/j.jsbmb.2017.01.021.

5. D. Swanson, R. Block, and S. A. Mousa, "Omega-3 Fatty Acids EPA and DHA: Health Benefits Throughout Life," *Advances in Nutrition* 3, no. 1 (January 2012): 1–7, https://doi.org/10.3945/an.111.000893.

6. J. M. Geleijnse, J. de Goede, and I. A. Brouwer, "Alpha-Linolenic Acid: Is It Essential to Cardiovascular Health?" *Current Atherosclerosis Reports* 12, no. 6 (November 2010): 359–67, https://doi.org/10.1007/s11883-010-0137-0.

7. N. Siriwardhana, N. S. Kalupahana, N. Moustaid-Moussa, "Health Benefits of n-3 Polyunsaturated Fatty Acids: Eicosapentaenoic Acid and Docosahexaenoic Acid," *Advances in Food and Nutrition Research* 65 (2012): 211–22, https://doi.org/10.1016/B978-0-12-416003-3.00013-5.

8. Siriwardhana et al., "Health Benefits of n-3 Polyunsaturated Fatty Acids," 211–22, https://doi.org/10.1016/B978-0-12-416003-3.00013-5.

9. A. P. Simopoulos, "The Importance of the Ratio of Omega-6/Omega-3 Essential Fatty Acids," *Biomedicine & Pharmacotherapy* 56, no. 8 (October 2002): 365–79.

10. P. M. Kris-Etherton, J. A. Grieger, and T. D. Etherton, "Dietary Reference Intakes for DHA and EPA," *Prostaglandins, Leukotrienes and Essential Fatty Acids* 81, no. 2–3 (August–September 2009): 99–104, https://doi.org/10.1016/j.plefa.2009.05.011.

11. W. W. Winder and D. G. Hardie, "AMP-Activated Protein Kinase, a Metabolic Master Switch: Possible Roles in Type 2 Diabetes," *American Journal of Physiology* 277, no. 1 (July 1999): E1–10, https://doi.org/10.1152/ajpendo.1999.277.1.E1.

12. H. Wang et al., "Metformin and Berberine, Two Versatile Drugs in Treatment of Common Metabolic Diseases," *Oncotarget* 9, no. 11 (2018): 10135–46, https://doi.org/10.18632/oncotarget.20807.

13. D. Townsend et al., "Epigallocatechin-3-Gallate Remodels Apolipoprotein A-I Amyloid Fibrils into Soluble Oligomers in the Presence of Heparin," *Journal of Biological Chemistry* 293 (2018): 12877–93, https://doi.org/10.1074/jbc.RA118.002038.

14. M. Lindefeldt et al., "The Ketogenic Diet Influences Taxonomic and Functional Composition of the Gut Microbiota in Children with Severe Epilepsy," *NPJ Biofilms Microbiomes* 5 (January 2019): 5, https://doi.org/10.1038/s41522-018-0073-2.

15. B. Kleessen et al., "Jerusalem Artichoke and Chicory Inulin in Bakery Products Affect Faecal Microbiota of Healthy Volunteers," *British Journal of Nutrition* 98, no. 3 (September 2007): 540–9.

16. D. Ríos-Covián et al., "Intestinal Short Chain Fatty Acids and Their Link with Diet and Human Health," *Frontiers in Microbiology* 7 (February 2016): 185, https://doi.org/10.3389/fmicb.2016.00185.

17. L. Samal et al., "Prebiotic Potential of Jerusalem Artichoke (*Helianthus tuberosus* L.) in Wistar Rats: Effects of Levels of Supplementation on Hindgut Fermentation, Intestinal Morphology, Blood Metabolites and Immune Response," *Journal of the Science of Food and Agriculture* 95, no. 8 (June 2015): 1689–96, https://doi.org/10.1002/jsfa.6873.

18. W. C. Chang et al., "Beneficial Effects of Soluble Dietary Jerusalem Artichoke (*Helianthus tuberosus*) in the Prevention of the Onset of Type 2 Diabetes and Non-Alcoholic Fatty Liver Disease in High-Fructose Diet-Fed Rats," *British Journal of Nutrition* 112, no. 5 (September 2014): 709–17, https://doi.org/10.1017/S0007114514001421.

19. R. Babiker et al., "Effect of Gum Arabic *(Acacia Senegal)* Supplementation on Visceral Adiposity Index (VAI) and Blood Pressure in Patients with Type 2 Diabetes Mellitus as Indicators of Cardiovascular Disease (CVD): A Randomized and Placebo-Controlled Clinical Trial," *Lipids in Health and Disease* 17, no. 1 (March 2018): 56, https://doi.org/10.1186/s12944-018-0711-y.

20. R. Babiker et al., "Effects of Gum Arabic Ingestion on Body Mass Index and Body Fat Percentage in Healthy Adult Females: Two-Arm Randomized, Placebo Controlled, Double-Blind Trial," *Nutrition Journal* 11 (December 2012): 111, https://doi.org/10.1186/1475-2891-11-111.

21. B. Upadhyaya et al., "Impact of Dietary Resistant Starch Type 4 on Human Gut Microbiota and Immunometabolic Functions," *Scientific Reports* 6 (June 2016): 28797, https://doi.org/10.1038/srep28797.

22. C. Cangiano et al., "Effects of Oral 5-Hydroxy-Tryptophan on Energy Intake and Macronutrient Selection in Non-Insulin Dependent Diabetic Patients," *International Journal of Obesity* 22, no. 7 (July 1998): 648–54.

23. K. Shaw, J. Turner, and C. Del Mar, "Tryptophan and 5-Hydroxytryptophan for Depression," *Cochrane Database of Systematic Reviews* no. 1 (January 2002): CD003198, https://doi.org/10.1002/14651858.CD003198.

24. F. Titus, "5-Hydroxytryptophan Versus Methysergide in the Prophylaxis of Migraine. Randomized clinical trial," *European Neurology* 25, no. 5 (1986): 327–9, https://doi.org/10.1159/000116030.

25. B. Kim, "Thyroid Hormone as a Determinant of Energy Expenditure and the Basal Metabolic Rate," Thyroid 18, no. 2 (February 2008): 141–4, https://doi.org/10.1089/thy.2007.0266.

26. D. Yagnik, V. Serafin, and A. J. Shah, "Antimicrobial Activity of Apple Cider Vinegar against *Escherichia coli*, *Staphylococcus aureus* and *Candida albicans*; Downregulating Cytokine and Microbial Protein Expression," 1732.

27. S. Sakakibara et al., "Acetic Acid Activates Hepatic AMPK and Reduces Hyperglycemia in Diabetic KK-A(y) Mice," *Biochemical and Biophysical Research Communications* 344, no. 2 (June 2006): 597–604, https://doi.org/ 10.1016/j.bbrc .2006.03.176.

28. H. Yamashita et al., "Improvement of Obesity and Glucose Tolerance by Acetate in Type 2 Diabetic Otsuka Long-Evans Tokushima Fatty (OLETF) Rats," *Bioscience, Biotechnology, and Biochemistry* 71, no. 5 (May 2007): 1236–43.

29. G. Frost et al., "The Short-Chain Fatty Acid Acetate Reduces Appetite Via a Central Homeostatic Mechanism," *Nature Communications* 5 (April 2014): 3611, https://doi.org/ 10.1038/ncomms4611.

# Chapter 7

1. The GBD 2015 Obesity Collaborators, "Health Effects of Overweight and Obesity in 195 Countries over 25 Years," *The New England Journal of Medicine* 377, no. 1 (July 2017): 13–27, https://doi.org/ 10.1056/NEJMoa161436.

2. G. W. Reed and J. O. Hill, "Measuring the Thermic Effect of Food," *The American Journal of Clinical Nutrition* 63, no. 2 (February 1996): 164–9, https://doi.org/10.1093/ajcn/63.2.164.

3. W. N. Stainsby and J. K. Barclay, "Exercise Metabolism: O2 Deficit, Steady Level O2 Uptake and O2 Uptake for Recovery," *Medicine & Science in Sports & Exercise* 2, no. 4 (Winter 1970): 177–81.

4. M. F. Leitzmann et al., "Physical Activity Recommendations and Decreased Risk of Mortality," *Archives of Internal Medicine* 167, no. 22 (December 2007): 2453–60, https://doi.org/ 10.1001/archinte.167.22.2453.

5. J. A. Levine, "Non-Exercise Activity Thermogenesis (NEAT)," *Best Practice & Research: Clinical Endocrinology & Metabolism* 16, no. 4 (December 2002): 679–702.

6. J. A. Levine, M. W. Vander Weg, and R. C. Klesges, "Increasing Non-Exercise Activity Thermogenesis: A NEAT Way to Increase Energy Expenditure in Your Patients," *Obesity Management* 2, no. 4 (September 2006): 146–151, https://doi .org/10.1089/obe.2006.2.146.

7. J. A. Levine, "Nonexercise Activity Thermogenesis—Liberating the Life-Force," *Journal of Internal Medicine* 262, no. 3 (September 2007): 273–87, https://doi.org/ 10.1111/j.1365-2796.2007.01842.x.

8. C. Tudor-Locke and D. R. Bassett, Jr., "How Many Steps/Day Are Enough? Preliminary Pedometer Indices for Public Health," *Sports Medicine* 34, no. 1 (January 2004): 1–8, https://doi.org/10.2165/00007256-200434010-00001.

9. A. Paoli et al., "Beyond Weight Loss: A Review of the Therapeutic Uses of Very-Low-Carbohydrate (Ketogenic) Diets," *European Journal of Clinical Nutrition* 67, no. 8 (August 2013): 789–96, https://doi.org/10.1038/ejcn.2013.116.

10. T. A. Lakka and D. E. Laaksonen, "Physical Activity in Prevention and Treatment of the Metabolic Syndrome," *Applied Physiology, Nutrition, and Metabolism* 32, no. 1 (February 2007): 76–88, https://doi.org/10.1139/h06-113.

11. J. Clarke and I. Janssen, "Is the Frequency of Weekly Moderate-To-Vigorous Physical Activity Associated with the Metabolic Syndrome in Canadian Adults?" *Applied Physiology, Nutrition, and Metabolism* 38, no. 7 (July 2013): 773–8, https://doi.org/10.1139/apnm-2013-0049.

12. C. H. Yang and D. E. Conroy, "Momentary Negative Affect Is Lower During Mindful Movement than While Sitting: An Experience Sampling Study," *Psychology of Sport and Exercise* 37 (July 2018): 109–116, https://doi.org/10.1016/ j.psychsport.2018.05.003.

13. M. Iwane et al., "Walking 10,000 Steps/Day or More Reduces Blood Pressure and Sympathetic Nerve Activity in Mild Essential Hypertension," *Hypertension Research* 23, no. 6 (November 2000): 573–80.

14. R. A. Rodrigues de Oliveira et al. "Association Between the Number of Daily Steps and the Cardiovascular Risk Factors in Basic Education Teachers," *The Journal of Sports Medicine and Physical Fitness* 58, no. 5 (May 2018): 714–20, https://doi.org/10.23736/S0022-4707.17.07330-3.

15. N. Yamamoto et al., "Daily Step Count and All-Cause Mortality in a Sample of Japanese Elderly People: A Cohort Study," *BMC Public Health* 18, no. 1 (April 2018): 540, https://doi.org/10.1186/s12889-018-5434-5.

16. I. M. Lee and D. M. Buchner, "The Importance of Walking to Public Health," *Medicine & Science in Sports & Exercise* 40, no. 7 (July 2008): S512–8, https://doi .org/10.1249/MSS.0b013e31817c65d0.

17. Catrine Tudor-Locke et al., "Step-Based Physical Activity Metrics and Cardiometabolic Risk," *Medicine & Science in Sports & Exercise* 49, no. 2 (February 2017): 283–91, https://doi.org/10.1249/MSS.0000000000001100.

18. Catrine Tudor-Locke et al., "How Many Steps/Day Are Enough? For Adults," *International Journal of Behavioral Nutrition and Physical Activity* 8 (July 2011): 79, https://doi.org/10.1186/1479-5868-8-79.

19. J. D. Pillay et al., "Steps That Count: Physical Activity Recommendations, Brisk Walking, and Steps Per Minute—How Do They Relate?" *Journal of Physical Activity and Health* 11, no. 3 (March 2014): 502–8, https://doi.org/10.1123/jpah.2012-0210.

20. W. L. Haskell et al., "Physical Activity and Public Health: Updated Recommendation for Adults from the American College of Sports Medicine and the American Heart Association," *Medicine & Science in Sports & Exercise* 39, no. 8 (August 2007): 1423–34, https://doi.org/10.1249/mss.0b013e3180616b27.

21. T. M. Eijsvogels and P. D. Thompson, "Exercise Is Medicine: At Any Dose?" *JAMA* 314, no. 18 (November 2015): 1915–6, https://doi.org/10.1001/jama.2015.10858.

22. K. Berczik et al., "Exercise Addiction: Symptoms, Diagnosis, Epidemiology, and Etiology," *Substance Use & Misuse* 47, no. 4 (March 2012): 403–17, https://doi.org/10.3109/10826084.2011.639120.

23. R. Foley and T. Kistemann, "Blue Space Geographies: Enabling Health in Place," *Health & Place* 35 (September 2015): 157–65, https://doi.org/10.1016/j.healthplace.2015.07.003.

24. C. Twohig-Bennett and A. Jones, "The Health Benefits of the Great Outdoors: A Systematic Review and Meta-Analysis of Greenspace Exposure and Health Outcomes," *Environmental Research* 166 (October 2018): 628–37, https://doi.org/10.1016/j.envres.2018.06.030.

25. A. H. Shadyab et al., "Associations of Accelerometer-Measured and Self-Reported Sedentary Time with Leukocyte Telomere Length in Older Women," *American Journal of Epidemiology* 185, no. 3 (February 2017): 172–84, https://doi.org/10.1093/aje/kww196.

26. University of California – Los Angeles, "Sitting Is Bad for Your Brain—Not Just Your Metabolism or Heart: Thinning in Brain Regions Important for Memory Linked to Sedentary Habits," *ScienceDaily*, April 12, 2018, https://www.sciencedaily.com/releases/2018/04/180412141014.htm.

27. L. Yang et al., "Trends in Sedentary Behavior Among the US Population, 2001–2016," *JAMA* 321, no. 16 (April 2019): 1587–97, https://doi.org/10.1001/jama.2019.3636.

28. F. Saeidifard et al., "Differences of Energy Expenditure While Sitting Versus Standing: A Systematic Review and Meta-Analysis," *European Journal of Preventive Cardiology* 5, no. 25 (March 2018): 522–38, https://doi.org/10.1177/2047487317752186.

29. M. L. Larouche et al., "Using Point-of-Choice Prompts to Reduce Sedentary Behavior in Sit-Stand Workstation Users," *Frontiers in Public Health* 6 (November 2018): 323, https://doi.org/10.3389/fpubh.2018.00323.

30. G. Hagger-Johnson et al., "Sitting Time, Fidgeting, and All-Cause Mortality in the UK Women's Cohort Study," *American Journal of Preventive Medicine* 50, no. 2 (February 2016): 154–60, https://doi.org/10.1016/j.amepre.2015.06.025.

31.  T. Morishima et al., "Prolonged Sitting-Induced Leg Endothelial Dysfunction Is Prevented by Fidgeting," *American Journal of Physiology: Heart and Circulatory Physiology* 311, no. 1 (July 2016): H177–82, https://doi.org/10.1152/ajpheart.00297.2016.

## Chapter 8

1.  T. A. Miller and M. R. Dimatteo, "Importance of Family/Social Support and Impact on Adherence to Diabetic Therapy," *Diabetes, Metabolic Syndrome and Obesity: Targets and Therapy* 2013, no. 6 (November 2013): 421–6, https://doi.org/10.2147/DMSO.S36368.

2.  H. G. Hers, "The Control of Glycogen Metabolism in the Liver," *Annual Review of Biochemistry* 45 (1976): 167–89, https://doi.org/10.1146/annurev.bi.45.070176.001123.

3.  T. Chang et al., "Inadequate Hydration, BMI, and Obesity Among US Adults: NHANES 2009–2012," *Annals of Family Medicine* 14, no. 4 (July/August 2016): 320–324, https://doi.org/10.1370/afm.1951.

4.  Institute of Medicine of the National Academies, *Dietary Reference Intakes for Water, Potassium, Sodium, Chloride, and Sulfate* (Washington, DC: The National Academies Press, 2005), www.nap.edu/read/10925/chapter/1.

5.  A. M. Johnstone et al., "Effects of a High-Protein Ketogenic Diet on Hunger, Appetite, and Weight Loss in Obese Men Feeding Ad Libitum," *The American Journal of Clinical Nutrition* 87, no. 1 (January 2008): 44–55, https://doi.org/10.1093/ajcn/87.1.44.

6.  L. E. Burke, J. Wang, and M. A. Sevick, "Self-Monitoring in Weight Loss: A Systematic Review of the Literature," *Journal of the Academy of Nutrition and Dietetics* 111, no. 1 (2011): 92–102, https://doi.org/10.1016/j.jada.2010.10.008.

7.  S. Henley and S. Misner, "Dietary Fiber," University of Arizona College of Agriculture, August 1999, http://mail.konjacfoods.com/fiber/fiberar.pdf.

8.  J. J. Otten, J. P. Hellwig, and L. D. Meyers, *Dietary Reference Intakes: The Essential Guide to Nutrient Requirements* (Washington, DC: The National Academies Press, 2006).

## Fat Fuel

1.  M. W. Bourassa et al., "Butyrate, Neuroepigenetics and the Gut Microbiome: Can a High Fiber Diet Improve Brain Health?" *Neuroscience Letters* 625 (2016): 56–63, https://doi.org/10.1016/j.neulet.2016.02.009.

## Fiber Feasts

1.  P. Ranasinghe et al., "Efficacy and Safety of 'True' Cinnamon (*Cinnamomum zeylanicum*) as a Pharmaceutical Agent in Diabetes: A Systematic Review and Meta-Analysis," *Diabetic Medicine* 29, no. 12 (December 2012): 1480–92, https://doi.org/10.1111/j.1464-5491.2012.03718.x.

2. L. Tavares et al., "Neuroprotective Effects of Digested Polyphenols from Wild Blackberry Species," *European Journal of Nutrition* 52, no. 1 (February 2013): 225–36, https://doi.org/ 10.1007/s00394-012-0307-7.

3. M. Lyu et al., "Balancing Herbal Medicine and Functional Food for Prevention and Treatment of Cardiometabolic Diseases through Modulating Gut Microbiota," *Frontiers in Microbiology* 8 (November 2017): 2146, https://doi.org/ 10.3389/fmicb.2017.02146.

## 'Biome Boosters

1. P. Suttiwan, P. Yuktanandana, and S. Ngamake, "Effectiveness of Essence of Chicken on Cognitive Function Improvement: A Randomized Controlled Clinical Trial," *Nutrients* 10, no. 7 (June 2018): 845, https://doi.org/10.3390/ nu10070845.

2. S. Parvez et al., "Probiotics and Their Fermented Food Products Are Beneficial for Health," *Journal of Applied Microbiology* 100, no. 6 (June 2006): 1171–85, https://doi.org/10.1111/j.1365-2672.2006.02963.x.

3. T. Hussain et al., "Oxidative Stress and Inflammation: What Polyphenols Can Do for Us?" *Oxidative Medicine and Cellular Longevity* 2016 (2016): 7432797, https://doi.org/10.1155/2016/7432797.

4. A. Costabile, "A double-blind, placebo-controlled, cross-over study to establish the bifidogenic effect of a very-long-chain inulin extracted from globe artichoke *(Cynara scolymus)* in healthy human subjects," *The British Journal of Nutrition* 104, no.7 (October 2010): 1007–17, https://doi.org/10.1017/S0007114510001571.

5. S. Manchali, K. N. C. Murthy, and B. S. Patil, "Crucial Facts about Health Benefits of Popular Cruciferous Vegetables," *Journal of Functional Foods* 4, no. 1 (January 2012): 94–106, https://doi.org/10.1016/j.jff.2011.08.004.

6. D. Y. Oh et al., "GPR120 Is an Omega-3 Fatty Acid Receptor Mediating Potent Anti-Inflammatory and Insulin-Sensitizing Effects," *Cell* 142, no. 5 (September 2010): 687–98, https://doi.org/10.1016/j.cell.2010.07.041.

7. Manchali et al., "Crucial Facts about Health Benefits of Popular Cruciferous Vegetables," 94–106, https://doi.org/10.1016/j.jff.2011.08.004.

8. A. Zeb, "Phenolic Profile and Antioxidant Potential of Wild Watercress *(Nasturtium officinale L.)*," *SpringerPlus* 4 (November 2015): 714, https://doi.org/ 10.1186/s40064-015-1514-5.

9. I. Ivanov, "Polyphenols Content and Antioxidant Activities of Taraxacum officinale F.H. Wigg (dandelion) leaves," *International Journal of Pharmacognosy and Phytochemical Research* 6, no. 4 (December 2014): 889–93.

10. N. Farmer, K. Touchton-Leonard, and A. Ross, "Psychosocial Benefits of Cooking Interventions: A Systematic Review," *Health Education & Behavior* 45, no. 2 (2018): 167–80, https://doi.org/10.1177/1090198117736352.

11. M. Mihic et al., "Nutritive quality of romanian hemp varieties *(Cannabis sativa L.)* with special focus on oil and metal contents of seeds," *Chemistry Central Journal* 6, no. 122 (October 2012), https://doi.org/10.1186/1752-153X-6-122.

12. G. A. Manganaris et al., "Berry Antioxidants: Small Fruits Providing Large Benefits," *Journal of the Science of Food & Agriculture* 94, no. 5 (March 2014): 825–33, https://doi.org/10.1002/jsfa.6432.

13. J. Volden et al., "Processing (Blanching, Boiling, Steaming) Effects on the Content of Glucosinolates and Antioxidant-Related Parameters in Cauliflower (*Brassica oleracea* L. ssp. *botrytis*)," *LWT - Food Science and Technology* 42, no. 1 (2009): 63–73, https://doi.org/10.1016/j.lwt.2008.05.018.

14. D. P. Cladis et al., "Fatty Acid Profiles of Commercially Available Finfish Fillets in the United States," *Lipids* 49, no. 10 (October 2014): 1005–18, https://doi.org/10.1007/s11745-014-3932-5.

15. B. M. Yashodhara et al., "Omega-3 Fatty Acids: A Comprehensive Review of Their Role in Health and Disease," *Postgraduate Medical Journal* 85, no. 1000 (February 2009): 84–90, https://doi.org/10.1136/pgmj.2008.073338.

16. Manchali et al., "Crucial Facts about Health Benefits of Popular Cruciferous Vegetables," 94–106, https://doi.org/10.1016/j.jff.2011.08.004.

17. M. F. McCarty, J. J. DiNicolantonio, and J. H. O'Keefe, "Capsaicin May Have Important Potential for Promoting Vascular and Metabolic Health," *Openheart* 2, no. 1 (June 2015): e000262, https://doi.org/10.1136/openhrt-2015-000262.

18. C. Stanton et al., "Probiotic cheese," *International Dairy Journal* 8, nos. 5–6 (May 1998) 8: 491–6.

19. Dreher and Davenport, "Hass Avocado Composition and Potential Health Effects," 738–50.

20. M. L. Garg et al., "Macadamia Nut Consumption Modulates Favourably Risk Factors for Coronary Artery Disease in Hypercholesterolemic Subjects," *Lipids* 42, no. 6 (June 2007): 583–7, https://doi.org/10.1007/s11745-007-3042-8.

21. A. N. Panche, A. D. Diwan, and S. R. Chandra, "Flavonoids: An Overview," *Journal of Nutritional Science* 5 (December 2016): e47, https://doi.org/10.1017/jns.2016.41.

22. S. K. Duckett et al., "Effects of Time on Feed on Beef Nutrient Composition," *Journal of Animal Science* 71, no. 8 (August 1993): 2079–88, https://doi.org/10.2527/1993.7182079x.

23. G. R. Gibson, "Dietary Modulation of the Human Gut Microflora Using the Prebiotics Oligofructose and Inulin," *The Journal of Nutrition* 129, no. 7 (July 1999): 1438S–41S, https://doi.org/10.1093/jn/129.7.1438S.

24. S. Buesing et al., "Vitamin B12 as a Treatment for Pain," *Pain Physician* 22, no. 1 (January 2019): E45–52.

25. R. Grzanna, L. Lindmark, and C. G. Frondoza, "Ginger—an Herbal Medicinal Product with Broad Anti-Inflammatory Actions," *Journal of Medicinal Food* 8, no. 2 (Summer 2005): 125–32, https://doi.org/10.1089/jmf.2005.8.125.

26. Panche et al., "Flavonoids: An Overview," e47, https://doi.org/10.1017/jns.2016.41.

27. S. Ghosh, S. Banerjee, P. C. Sil, "The Beneficial Role of Curcumin on Inflammation, Diabetes and Neurodegenerative Disease: A Recent Update," *Food and Chemical Toxicology* 83 (September 2015): 111–24, https://doi.org/10.1016/j.fct.2015.05.022.

28. P. C. K. Cheung, "The Nutritional and Health Benefits of Mushrooms," *Nutrition Bulletin* 35, no. 4 (December 2010): 292–9, https://doi.org/10.1111/j.1467-3010.2010.01859.x.

29. Manchali et al., "Crucial Facts about Health Benefits of Popular Cruciferous Vegetables," 94–106, https://doi.org/10.1016/j.jff.2011.08.004.

30. J. K. Kim and S. U. Park, "Current Potential Health Benefits of Sulforaphane," *EXCLI Journal* 15 (October 2016): 571–7, https://doi.org/10.17179/excli2016-485.

31. D. L. McKay et al., "A Pecan-Rich Diet Improves Cardiometabolic Risk Factors in Overweight and Obese Adults: A Randomized Controlled Trial," *Nutrients* 10, no. 3 (March 2018): 339, https://doi.org/10.3390/nu10030339.

32. M. Imran, M. S. Butt, H. A. R. Suleria, "*Capsicum annuum* Bioactive Compounds: Health Promotion Perspectives," in *Bioactive Molecules in Food, Reference Series in Phytochemistry*, eds. J. M. Mérillon and K. Ramawat (Springer, Cham: 2018).

33. A. Zarfeshany, S. Asgary, S. H. Javanmard, "Potent Health Effects of Pomegranate," *Advanced Biomedical Resarch* 3 (March 2014): 100, https://doi.org/10.4103/2277-9175.129371.

34. F. Giampieri et al., "The Strawberry: Composition, Nutritional Quality, and Impact on Human Health," *Nutrition* 28, no. 1 (January 2012): 9–19, https://doi.org/10.1016/j.nut.2011.08.009.

35. A. B. Kunnumakkara et al., "Chronic Diseases, Inflammation, and Spices: How Are They Linked?" *Journal of Translational Medicine* 16, no. 1 (January 2018): 14, https://doi.org/10.1186/s12967-018-1381-2.

# CraverTamers

1. M. Ibern-Gómez et al., "Resveratrol and Piceid Levels in Natural and Blended Peanut Butters," *Journal of Agricultural and Food Chemistry* 48, no. 12 (December 2000): 6352–4, https://doi.org/10.1021/jf000786k.

2. R. Latif, "Chocolate/Cocoa and Human Health: A Review," *The Netherlands Journal of Medicine* 71, no. 2 (March 2013): 63–8.

3. L. Kaume, L. R. Howard, and L. Devareddy, "The Blackberry Fruit: A Review on Its Composition and Chemistry, Metabolism and Bioavailability, and Health Benefits," *Journal of Agricultural and Food Chemistry* 60, no. 23 (June 2012): 5716–27, https://doi.org/10.1021/jf203318p.

4. N. Narang and W. Jiraungkoorskul, "Anticancer Activity of Key Lime, *Citrus aurantifolia*," *Pharmacognosy Review* 10, no. 20 (2016): 118–22, https://doi.org/10.4103/0973-7847.194043.

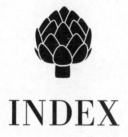

# INDEX

NOTE: Page references in *italics* refer to tables.

## Q

## R

## S

# ACKNOWLEDGMENTS

From my first interview with Dr. Jeff Bland, the father of functional medicine, for *The Real Skinny on Fat* docuseries, I knew everyone who watched and learned from it would have the knowledge and power to transform their own health, just as I had. With more than 70 world-renowned doctors, scientists, and other leading health experts teaching us about our health, I was put on the path to write *High Fiber Keto*. I am grateful to everyone who helped make this book a reality.

First, a huge thank you to each and every expert who generously contributed to *The Real Skinny on Fat*:

| | |
|---|---|
| Brooke Alpert, R.D. | Diana Blank |
| L. J. Amaral, R.D. | Michael Breus, Ph.D. |
| Stephen Anton, Ph.D. | Zach Bush, M.D. |
| Joseph Antoun, M.D. | James Chestnut, M.S., D.C. |
| Toni Bark, M.D. | Don Clum, D.C. |
| Franklin Becker | Dominic D'Agostino, Ph.D. |
| Alvin Berger, Ph.D. | Thomas Delauer |
| Jeff Bland, M.D. | William Troy Donahoo, M.D. |

Tanya Dorff, M.D.

William Dunn, Ph.D.

Erin Elizabeth

Dendy Engleman, M.D.

Udo Erasmus, Ph.D.

Kenneth Ford, Ph.D.

Jason Fung, M.D.

Felice Gersh, M.D.

Ben Greenfield

Paul Grewal, M.D.

Steven Gundry, M.D.

John Hardy

Randy Hartnell

Heather Hausenblas, Ph.D.

Jennifer Hays-Grudo, Ph.D.

Bryan Haycock, Ph.D.

Mike Hockenberry

Kurt Hong, M.D.

Mark Hyman, M.D.

Miriam Kalamian

Joel Khan, M.D.

Amy Killen, M.D.

Frank Lipman, M.D.

Gunnar Lovelace

Max Lugavere

Mindy Mackay-Swenson

Dori Madsen, personal trainer

Drew Manning

Christine Maren, osteopathic physician

Joe Maroon, M.D.

Tami Meraglia, M.D.

Joe Mercola, D.O.

Steve Morgan

Jeffrey Morrison, M.D.

Francis Murphy, D.C.

Mary Newport, M.D.

Angela Poff, Ph.D.

Dan Pompa, D.C.

Kellyann Petrucci, M.S., N.D.

Megan Ramos

Kendell Reichhart

David E. Root, physician

Thomas Seyfried, Ph.D.

Christopher Shade, Ph.D.

Cate Shanahan, M.D.

Mark Sisson

Jaclyn Sklaver, personal trainer

Kathy Smith

Kris Smith, M.D.

Jeff Spencer

Russell Swerdlow, M.D.

Nina Teicholz

Jenny Thompson

Shawn Wells, R.D.

Montel Williams

Beth Zupec-Kania, R.D.N.

I want to also thank the team of doctors, scientists, study participants, writers, and everyone else who helped me bring *High Fiber Keto* to life. I could not have done it without your expert minds—the world's best thinkers and researchers—who spend their days in the trenches seeking and finding answers. We are deeply indebted to all of you. Your explorations and dedication to your work are changing the world.

To my agent, Celeste Fine, and the team at Park & Fine Literary and Media (Sarah Passick, Anna Petkovich, and John Maas), you believed in my vision five years ago, which led to my first book, *Glow15*.

Through its creation and on to my dream for *High Fiber Keto*, you have offered your kindness and patience and continue to guide me on this adventure.

To the entire team at Hay House: Reid Tracy, Anne Barthel, Lisa Cheng, Patty Gift, Tricia Breidenthal, Lindsay McGinty, Alexandra Israel, Cathy Veloskey . . . Thank you for your incredible intellect and clear vision for our reader. Your deep support has been inspiring and appreciated.

To clinical nutritionist Lizzy Swick, M.S., R.D.N., your beautiful work has been invaluable. Thank you for your recipes and, more importantly, your unwavering commitment to this project.

To the women who participated in our study, I cannot thank you enough for your willingness to commit to your new lifestyles. And your eagerness to share your successes with the world has rewarded us all. Thank you for being the pioneers on this journey.

To Catherine Saenz, Ph.D., R.D., CSCS, thank you for your tireless work with the participants in our clinical study and for helping us show the world the amazing benefits of a high-fiber keto diet. Your dedication to the study group, your insight, and your kind support will always be remembered and deeply appreciated.

To Heather Hausenblas, Ph.D., thank you for your commitment to bringing our study together and to the women who entrusted us with their health and well-being. Your leadership, compassion, and support helped shape an outcome that will inspire so many more women to live their best lives.

To Stephen Anton, Ph.D., from *The Real Skinny on Fat* to *Glow15* to *High Fiber Keto* and everything in between, you have been a bright light of both expertise and inspiration.

To Sara Burke, Ph.D., thank you for sharing your vast knowledge about the relationship of our amazing brains to our overall health and how a ketogenic diet optimizes our performance. You have helped many people cut carbohydrates and maximize their mental performance. Your brain is an inspiration to all of us.

To Dr. Dana Cohen, thank you for sharing your wisdom about the deeper science of hydration that goes far beyond what most of us know about the importance and role of water in our bodies. Your exciting work is so appreciated.

To Dominic D'Agostino, Ph.D., this book would not be complete without your insights about ketones and their effect on our bodies. Thanks to you, we better understand how to use fat as energy and optimize our metabolic power. It is no surprise that you are known as the "King of Keto."

To Dr. Felice Gersh, board-certified OB/GYN, thank you for your nonstop energy, ideas, support, and inspiration. You are an encyclopedia of women's health, and your wisdom has informed, inspired, and improved countless lives. Thank you for always being there.

To Dr. Victoria Gershuni, thank you for providing your expertise about the microbiome, the keto diet, and how to eat for ketogenic success. Your time and knowledge made this a better book.

To Dr. Michael Hoaglin, thank you for your significant contributions to this and other projects. Your depth and breadth of knowledge about the microbiome and the benefits of a happy gut cannot be overstated.

To Dr. Erika Schwartz, thank you for your energy and your expertise on the importance of a healthy hormone balance. Your larger-than-life commitment to diet, exercise, and work-life balance distills the importance of overall well-being as a standard-bearer for good hormonal health. You are truly an inspiration.

To Brittanie Volk, Ph.D., R.D., your work is making the world a better place. You have already affected thousands of lives, with many more to come. Thank you for your guidance and caution in keeping us all in dietary lanes, especially at times when we should walk instead of run. You have taught us patience with the process that ensures long-term success.

To Beth Zupec-Kania, R.D.N., C.D., you are a nutritional ketosis superhero. Your understanding of our relationship with food is powerful and motivating. Thank you for your incredibly deep knowledge that brings to life the "little details" that are catalysts for great change.

To Myatt Murphy, thank you for the countless hours that took this book from a dream to a reality. You are an impressively talented writer who brings words, ideas, and important information to life in meaningful ways that serve us all so well.

To Ted Spiker, thank you for your time, energy, and enthusiasm for this book. You are a storyteller extraordinaire. Your writing paints pictures and helps us imagine information in new and exciting ways.

To Elayna Rexrode, thank you for your enduring devotion to all that we do. You keep us all on track and make it possible for us to accomplish so much. We could not do it without you.

To Bridget Grogan, thank you for bringing your perspective and truly meaningful ideas to the table. Your insights and feedback are deeply appreciated.

To all the University of Florida and University of Tennessee students who spent many months with us working on this book, thank you for your hard work, enthusiasm, new ideas, and optimism. You are talented, smart, and engaging.

Most importantly, thank you to my family, for the love, support, and time that you gave me through this second book adventure. You are my foundation, my inspiration, and my heart. I never would have had the opportunity to share this book with the world without all that each of you has given me.

To my parents for giving me such an incredible gift in life. It was as a child when you so brilliantly instilled in me a healthy lifestyle that has taken me this far, despite my personal health challenges. You are the foundation for the principles I am so deeply committed to and so honored to share in this book. I am proud of that, and I'm proud to be your daughter.

# ABOUT THE AUTHOR

**Naomi Whittel** is an entrepreneur, a leading nutritional expert, and the *New York Times* best-selling author of *Glow15*. She has made it her mission to better the lives of women by empowering them to take control of their health and providing them the opportunity to not just survive, but to thrive. A leader and innovator in the health and wellness industry, Naomi has two decades of experience in developing and managing sustainable companies. Naomi and her brands have been the recipients of the 2012 Business Achievement Award from *Nutrition Business Journal*, a Gold Stevie Award for Female Executive of the Year, and the Ernst and Young Entrepreneur of the Year Award. Named by *Prevention* as a leading female innovator in the natural products industry, Naomi is an advocate of clean and safe nutrition. Her story and products have been lauded by *The Wall Street Journal*, *Vogue*, *ELLE*, *Harper's Bazaar*, *ABC News*, PBS, *InStyle*, *The View*, *The Doctors*, *The Dr. Oz Show*, *SHAPE*, *Good Morning America*, and the *TODAY* show. Naomi is a mother of four and lives in Florida.

Join Naomi on her journey to a better life at www.naomiwhittel.com.

@NaomiWhittel   @naomiwhittel   @naomiwhittel   @NaomiWhittel   naomiwhittel

# Hay House Titles of Related Interest